D0598313

a guide to

homeopathy

a guide to
homeopathy

Andrew James

p

This is a Parragon Publishing Book

First published in 2002

Parragon Publishing

Queen Street House

4 Queen Street

Bath BA1 1HE, UK

ISBN: 0–75257–784–0

Printed in China

Produced by the Bridgewater Book Company Ltd

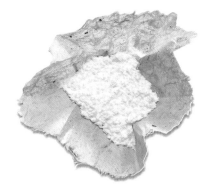

NOTE

Self-diagnosis and self-treatment for serious or long-term problems is not recommended. You should consult a medical professional or qualified practitioner. Seek professional advice before undertaking a course of self-treatment while you are undergoing a prescribed course of medical treatment. If your symptoms persist, seek medical advice.

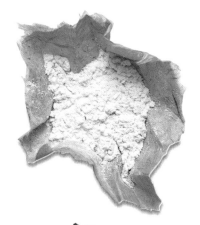

DEDICATION

This book is dedicated to Tom and Mary.

ACKNOWLEDGMENTS

The publishers wish to thank the following for the use of pictures:

A–Z Botanical Collection Ltd: 47t, 50t, 53t; *Jon Arnold Images* (www.jonarnold.com): 54b; *Corbis UK Ltd*: 8, 25t, 28t, 29b, 32t, 33t, 52t, 59t; *Getty Images*: 12r, 19b, 24b, 32b; *Natural History Museum Picture Library, London*: 43t; *NHPA*: 30t; *Science Photo Library*: 38b, 39t, 40b, 45t, 51t, 54t, 55t, 59b; *Harry Smith Horticultural Photographic Collection*: 46t, 57t.

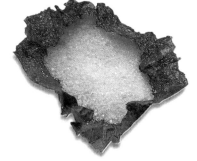

contents

Introduction

Homeopathy is one of many alternative and complementary therapies available today. Such therapies take a holistic approach to the treatment of patients. The word "holistic" is taken from the Greek word "holos" meaning "whole." The idea is that the person is treated as a whole, with every aspect of them—physical, emotional, and mental—being taken into account when selecting a remedy.

The purpose of this book is to introduce and describe the effects of the most common homeopathic remedies, enabling the reader to choose a remedy for the

Your doctor can refer you to a trained homeopath or another medical doctor who uses homeopathic treatments.

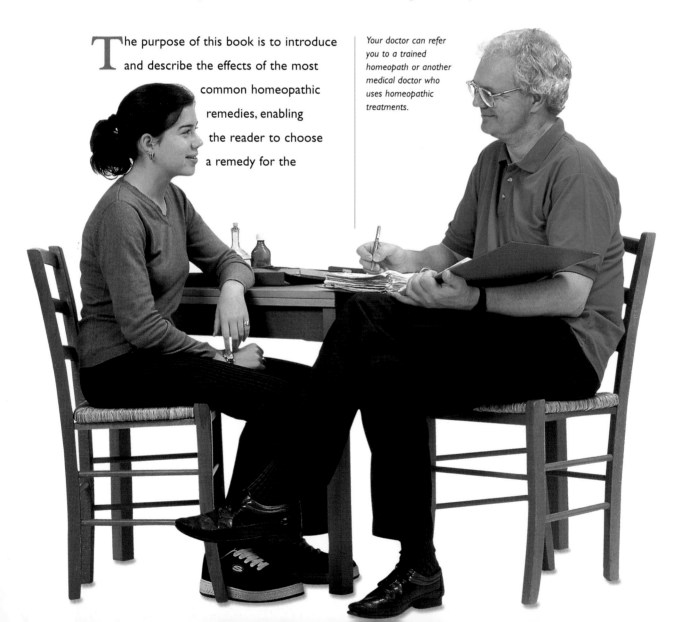

self-treatment of many common ailments, or to use them to complement conventional treatment. It should be stressed, however, that using this book for self-treatment should not replace conventional medicine. If you are concerned about your health, you should visit your doctor for a diagnosis before prescribing yourself any of the remedies. If you are currently under medical supervision, or are on a prescribed course of treatment, then check with your doctor or consultant before self-treating.

Although this book is a good way to begin self-treatment with homeopathy, it is worth noting that other forms of homeopathic treatment are also available.

Some hospitals offer homeopathic treatments from medically qualified doctors. Talk to your personal physician for referral. There are also medical doctors who are trained in homeopathy who work from their own practices, as well as non-medically qualified homeopaths who work in the same way. Some health care providers offer cover for homeopathic referral and treatment; check what is offered by your company.

Homeopathy has grown in popularity in recent years, and main street pharmacies now sell a large selection of homeopathic medicines. Some pharmacists are also trained in homeopathic pharmacy, so they may be able

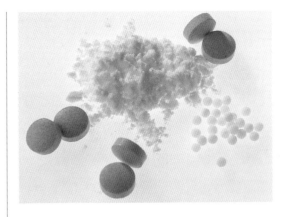

Today, homeopathic remedies are widely available. Many main street pharmacies stock a range of homeopathic medicines.

to help you choose a remedy. General stores, health food stores, airports, mail order, and internet companies also stock many of the most common remedies, so your chosen remedy should be easy to obtain.

Minor ailments such as colds can be successfully treated using homeopathy at home.

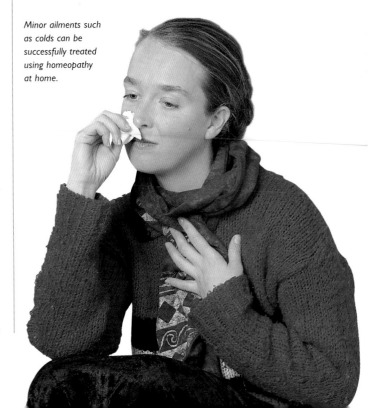

What is Homeopathy?

Homeopathy uses dilute substances to stimulate the body's healing power. Its basic principle is treat "like with like." This involves treating a patient's symptoms with minute amounts of a substance that would cause similar symptoms in a healthy person. This practice contrasts with conventional allopathic medicine, where treating "like with opposite" prevails; that is, a disease is treated with a substance that opposes it.

The first person to practice the healing principle of treating "like with like" was Greek physician Hippocrates (c.460–377BCE). His method went against the thinking of the time, which held that the gods were the main force behind a disease, and that a cure could be found by treating with a substance that had an opposite effect in a healthy person.

German doctor Samuel Hahnemann (1755–1843) was the modern-day founder of homeopathy. He proved the principle of "like curing like" with his experiments with quinine, known to be an effective treatment for malaria. He found he developed malarial symptoms after taking doses of quinine (he was otherwise in good health). These effects lasted hours after each dose.

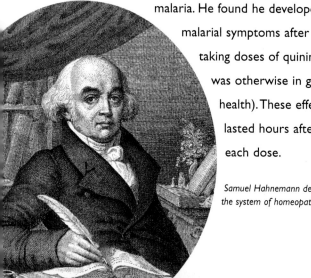

Samuel Hahnemann devised the system of homeopathy.

He tested other substances in the same way, in a process known as "proving." He "proved" more than 100 homeopathic remedies in his lifetime, publishing his findings in "The Organon of Rational Medicine" in 1811. He believed that the remedies worked by activating a person's "vital force," that is, the body's own healing potential. Having conducted tests on many volunteers, he came to realize the importance of taking into account the personality traits of each person receiving the treatment. He found that particular "types" of people manifested different symptoms to the same disease and so required treatment with different remedies in accordance with their "type."

American doctor James Tyler Kent (1849–1943) furthered Hahnemann's work on the different "types" of people and the matching of a remedy to their emotional and physical characteristics. These "types" became known as "constitutional types."

Remedy Dilution and Potentization

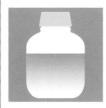
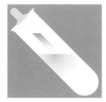
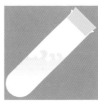
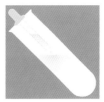
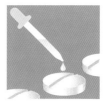

The mother tincture is prepared from the source material.

One drop of the tincture is diluted with 99 drops of alcohol and water.

The remedy is then succussed. This makes the 1c potency.

Using the 1c potency, the process is then repeated to reach the required potency.

A few drops are added to lactose tablets.

Homeopathic remedies

Remedies can be made from many different substances. The most common sources are flowers, plants, roots, trees, poisons, minerals, and metals. Certain insects are also used.

Hahnemann used the smallest possible amount of a substance to trigger a healing effect. This was to minimize side effects. He realized that the more a substance was diluted, the better the results, provided it was also vigorously shaken (in a process known as succussion) at each stage of dilution. Counter-intuitive though it seems, the less of the original substance that remained in the remedy, the greater its potency and effectiveness.

The process of diluting a remedy to render it effective is called potentization. First an alcohol/water extract is made from the substance. This is the mother tincture. The extract is diluted to the required potency. The main potencies are denoted by x, c, and m: x means the remedy has been diluted one part mother tincture in 9 drops of water; c means one part of mother tincture in 99 drops of water; and m means one part of mother tincture in 999 drops of water. A 1c potency is one part in 99 parts of water. A 2c potency is created by taking one part of the previous dilution (i.e., the 1c potency) and diluting it in 99 parts of water. The most common potencies used are 6c, 12c, and 30c.

Once the required potency is reached, a few drops of the substance are applied to lactose (milk sugar) tablets. The tablets must be kept dry and away from direct sunlight.

For the purposes of self-treatment as detailed here, it is suggested that the 30c potencies are used, as these are commonly available. To obtain the best results, consult a homeopath. They may prescribe higher potencies depending on the initial consultation and the presenting problem. This is particularly the case if the ailment has a strong emotional or mental aspect.

Using the Remedies

When taking the remedies orally it is possible to choose from several mediums that are available from a homeopathic pharmacy or supplier. The tablets also can often be found in a main street pharmacy or health store.

Tablets

These are the most readily available form. The tablets should be sucked or lightly chewed until they dissolve completely. This usually takes several minutes. Tablets are ideal for adults and older children.

Soft Tablets

These dissolve instantly on the tongue. They are ideal for young children, babies, and for adults who are impatient and do not want to spend time sucking or chewing.

Pillules

These are small, round, hard pills. They can take longer to dissolve in the mouth than ordinary tablets. This form is often found in homeopathic first aid kits because they are smaller than the tablets and fit easily into a smaller container.

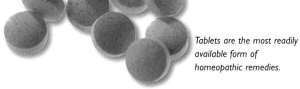

Tablets are the most readily available form of homeopathic remedies.

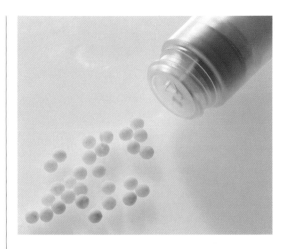

Pillules are small tablets that are dissolved slowly in the mouth. They are useful for homeopathic first aid kits.

Powders

Powders are usually prescribed by homeopaths for a single dose or several-dose treatment of a higher potency remedy (e.g. 200c or over, or 1m and over). They are supplied wrapped in paper and, like soft tablets, dissolve instantly on the tongue. It is possible simply to crush a tablet to make a powder by folding it in paper and hitting it with the back of a metal spoon. The powder can then be held in the paper, made into a funnel shape and poured into the mouth

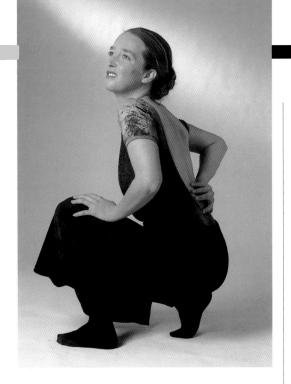

Back pain is a chronic condition that can be treated by taking several tablets a day.

for quick absorption. This method can be used in a first aid situation to administer a dose to young children or babies, or to children who refuse to take the tablets.

Frequency of Treatment

Once you have chosen a remedy, the next consideration is how often to take it. The main distinction is between acute and chronic conditions (acute illnesses have a rapid onset and short duration, whereas chronic conditions are of long duration and often gradual onset). For an acute condition such as an injury or a stomach upset, take one tablet every one to two hours for the first six doses (you can take fewer if the condition is relieved before this). If the condition does not improve

after six doses, continue with one tablet two or three times a day until the symptoms are relieved. Once there is improvement, stop taking the remedy immediately.

If the condition is chronic, such as irritable bowel syndrome, chronic fatigue syndrome, arthritis or depression, then one tablet should be taken twice a day until the condition has improved. Once the condition is relieved, stop the treatment immediately.

Stopping the treatment as soon as the condition improves may seem strange, because conventional medicines, such as antibiotics, often require the whole course to be completed. However, in homeopathy, it is of no benefit to continue a treatment once the condition improves.

If you notice no improvement from a remedy after giving it sufficient time to work, or notice only a very minor improvement, it is worth trying another remedy. Always take into account your constitutional type, if possible. The selection of remedies often involves some trial and error.

A bad cold is an acute condition that can be treated by taking a tablet every 1–2 hours.

Constitutional Types

Homeopathy treats the individual as a whole, taking into account physical, emotional, and mental states as well as disease or ailment. Knowing a person's constitutional type offers insight into the best remedy for them. This is particularly important, because two people suffering from the same problem may have different symptoms. They may find that different modalities (influences) improve or worsen their condition. Therefore, they may need to be treated with different remedies, despite having the same illness.

Mental and emotional factors of constitutional types are taken into consideration when prescribing. These include such matters as the individual's fears and anxieties—for example, whether they have a fear of animals, spiders, the dark, thunderstorms, loneliness, robbery, attack, failure, death or poisoning. It also takes into account an individual's temperament—whether they tend to be tearful, happy, sad, confident, lazy, perfectionist, mild, gentle, caring, optimistic, irritable, aggressive or spiteful. Then we need to examine whether certain factors affect the

Knowing a person's constitutional type can provide a valuable insight into their problem.

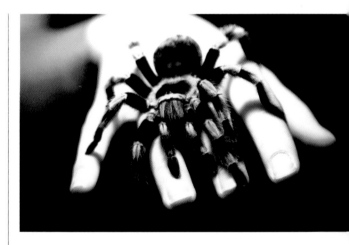

Knowing a person's fears and anxieties helps to reveal the emotional and mental state of the individual.

individual and whether they have an effect on the condition itself. For example, how do they respond to noise? Does music bring on emotional reactions? Are they bright and alert in the morning or dull and unresponsive? Do they like their own company or prefer to be with others? Do they prefer hot or cold weather? Do they prefer dry or wet atmospheres? Do they talk to others about problems or keep themselves to themselves? Do they have strong likes and dislikes for food and drinks?

Physical factors are also important. These aspects include whether the patient is tall or short; fat or thin; long-limbed; under- or overweight. Do they have dark rings under the eyes? What is their hair and eye color? Do they have thick, curly or thin hair? What is their skin texture? Preferred type of clothing? Is their manner of dress formal or casual? Do they have frown lines?

Once you have discerned someone's constitutional type, it is easier to select the most appropriate remedy. For example, consider a person who is suffering from a sore throat and cold. The best remedy for the physical symptoms of a sore throat and cold is remedy A, B or C. The best remedy for the emotional aspects of the person with the sore throat and cold is either remedy B or C. The best remedy according to the person's constitution is remedy B. Therefore, remedy B is likely to be most effective.

It is not essential to calculate the remedy in this way—prescribing remedy A based on the physical symptoms only will have some effect— but the best effect would be remedy B, because it fits all aspects for that individual.

Some of the main constitutional types are outlined on the next few pages.

The Argent. Nit. Type

Appearance: Pale complexion. Looks older than actual age, due to worry and tension.

Mental and emotional aspects: Cheerful and impressionable. Often anxious and worried. Always in a hurry and can be impulsive. Finds it difficult to control emotions. Readily laughs, cries, and loses temper. Quick-thinking and good at solving problems. Tends to be extraverted in order to hide true feelings.

Physical weaknesses: Nervous system. Digestive system. Eyes. Ailments tend to be left-sided.

Dietary factors: Likes chocolates, sweets, salt, and cheese. Dislikes chilled foods.

The Argent. nit. child: Always moving around and never wants to sit still. Prone to nervousness and can experience upset stomach when stressed. May react badly to new situations such as moving school. Can be prone to insomnia due to anxiety. Prone to bedwetting.

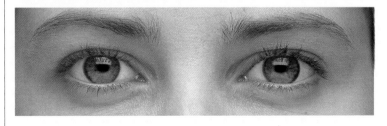

Argent. nit. types tend to have weak mucous membranes in their eyes.

The Arsen. Alb. Type

Appearance: Usually thin or slim. Often well groomed and "stylish." Fine facial features with delicate, sensitive skin. Frown lines can appear on the forehead.

Mental and emotional aspects: Restless person. Perfectionist at work and at home. Can be critical and intolerant. Strong opinions. Can have a deep fear of being alone. Obsessive-compulsive behavior, in particular involving cleanliness and "tidying up"; this can hide a hoarding mentality. Can pull out of plans and projects early if they think it is not going to work out 100%.

Warm drinks and sweet foods are favored by the Arsen. alb. type.

Pessimistic in nature, with a need to receive constant reassurance.

Physical weakness: Digestive system. Skin. Respiratory system (asthma, coughs, and colds).

Dietary factors: Likes fatty foods, warm food and drinks, in particular coffee, sweets, alcohol, and sour-tasting foods. Dislikes large amount of fluid.

The Arsen. alb. child: Highly sensitive and "highly strung." Easily upset by loud noise. Becomes tired and exhausted after periods of exertion. Suffers nightmares due to very active imagination. Increasingly physically and mentally agile with age. Can worry too much about parents' well-being. Keeps room neat and tidy. Does not like mess or getting messy.

The Calc. Carb. Type

Appearance: Overweight or gains weight easily. Sluggish, bloated, and tired in appearance. May have poor posture.

Mental and emotional aspects: Impressionable. Sensitive and quiet. May become withdrawn due to a deep fear of failure. Can dwell too much on a particular problem. May be greatly upset by cruelty to animals or children. Needs motivation to succeed in tasks. Can be prone to mild depression when unwell. Reassurance helps to improve condition.

Physical weaknesses: Ears, nose, and throat. Skeletal system (may manifest in backache). Digestive system: may be prone to irritable bowel syndrome and bloatedness. Skin. Teeth. Exhaustion; prone to chronic fatigue syndrome. Prone to depression.

Dietary factors: Likes dairy products, eggs, sweets, salt, desserts, chocolate, carbohydrates, iced drinks, and ice-cream. Dislikes fatty meat, boiled food, and boiled milk.

The Calc. carb. child: Plump and overweight. Placid and calm. Complexion often pale. Slow to walk and talk and teeth are slow to develop. Can fall over easily. Scared of the dark and prone to waking up because of nightmares. Often lazy and may need encouragement with schoolwork as gives up easily.

The ears, nose, and throat are all weak areas of the Calc. carb. type.

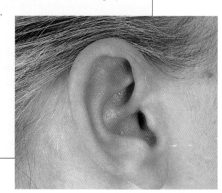

The Graphites Type

Appearance: Prone to being overweight and has a large appetite. Blushes easily. Can have a rugged, windswept appearance. May have rough, dry skin that can crack and flake easily. Dry hair, usually dark in color. Flaky scalp.

Mental and emotional aspects: A plodder— takes time to work things out and solve problems. Deep concentration on a task can cause irritability. Unwilling to change attitudes and routines. Not best first thing in the morning. Prone to mood swings. Can become tearful and despondent and then impatient.

Physical weaknesses: Skin. Nails. Slow metabolic rate. Common ailments may include soreness in the corners of the mouth, exhaustion, bad breath, nose bleeds, styes, and travel sickness.

Dietary factors: Likes sour and savory foods, cool drinks. Dislikes sweet foods, salt, seafood, hot drinks.

The Graphites child: Feels the cold and gets chilled very quickly. Timid, hesitant, and anxious. Does not like long periods of travel, as often suffers from travel sickness.

The Graphites type likes savory foods, such as salads or vegetables, rather than sweets and desserts.

The Ignatia Type

Appearance: Slim build. Prone to dark circles under the eyes. May have a tired, drawn expression and involuntary twitching of the eyes and mouth. Dry lips. Hair is of a dark to medium color. Sighs a lot.

Mental and emotional aspects: The most highly strung of the constitutional types. Tendency to rapid and extreme mood swings. Can switch quickly from depression to joy and from tears to laughter. Prone to suppressing grief. May find it difficult to end relationships and perceive this to be a weakness. Addictions to nicotine and caffeine are common.

Physical weaknesses: Nervous system. Emotional trauma may be the cause of any number of physical problems. Common problems include hysterical grief over bereavement, leading to depression, headaches, sore throats, coughs and colds, constipation, twitching, and grinding of teeth.

Dietary factors: Likes coffee (although it may not agree with them), sour and savory foods, dairy products, carbohydrates. Dislikes sweet foods.

The Ignatia child: Highly strung. Excitable and sensitive. Finds it difficult to perform under stress. Finds separation or divorce of parents very hard to deal with, leading to outbursts of anger, crying, and poor performance at school. Prefers company to being alone. May suffer with headaches, coughs, sore throats. Responds well to reassurance.

Dairy foods are popular with the Ignatia type.

The Lachesis Type

Appearance: May look bloated or lean. Strong, fixed expression. Complexion usually pale and prone to slight freckles. Strong and staring eyes. Can lick the lips a lot.

Mental and emotional aspects: Very ambitious. Highly creative. Mind can become crowded with thoughts. Jealous and possessive. Talkative. Can be sensitive to noise. If religious, is prone to view self as sinful. Can be suspicious of strangers.

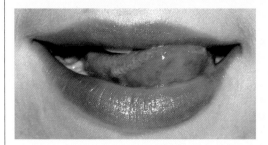

Physical weaknesses: Circulation. Nervous system. Common problems include varicose veins, hyperactivity, menopausal problems, sore throats, and asthma, disturbed sleep and insomnia, palpitations, and panic attacks. Prone to left-sided problems. Physical problems made worse when trying to sleep or remain still.

Dietary factors: Likes coffee, alcohol, seafood, cool drinks, sour and savory food, and carbohydrates. Dislikes sweet drinks.

The Lachesis child: Spiteful, possessive, and can be hurtful to peers. Hyperactive. Jealous of siblings, particularly newly born. Prone to nightmares. May be prone to ADHD (attention deficit and hyperactivity disorder).

Lachesis types have a tendency to lick their top lip.

The Lycopodium Type

Appearance: Tall and lean. Worry and frown lines on the forehead. Can look older than their actual years. Facial twitches. Thinning hair in men. Dislikes wearing tight clothing.

Mental and emotional aspects: Prone to exaggeration. Can create a drama over minor matters. Insecure and hates change. Avoids commitment. Anxious of challenging events. Strong fear of being alone and of the dark. Forgetful. Finds small mistakes disproportionately irritating. Hates being contradicted.

Physical weakness: Common problems include digestive disorders, kidney stones, prostate problems, headaches, sore throats, male-pattern baldness, and alopecia. May be prone to chronic fatigue syndrome.

Right-sided problems are more prevalent.

Dietary factors: Likes sweet foods, warm drinks, onions, garlic, and seafood. Dislikes cheese and strongly flavored meats.

The Lycopodium child: Basically insecure and shy, although can be bossy and dominant with other children. Likes to be indoors rather than doing outdoor pursuits. Likes to read and is conscientious and good academically.

The hairline of Lycopodium men recedes early and they may become prematurely gray or bald.

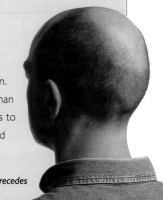

The Merc. Sol. Type

Appearance: Medium build. Skin on the face may be shiny or moist due to perspiration, with a gray translucent look. Hair color may be fair to medium.

Mental and emotional aspects: May have an inner battle with emotions. Resentment, anxiety, and lack of trust in others may cause feelings of insecurity. Dislikes criticism that is directed at self or taking orders from others. May explode with rage and anger.

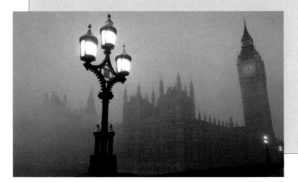

Memory may become poor with age and thought patterns may become muddled later in life.

Physical weaknesses: Common problems include sore throat; swelling of glands; exhaustion. Skin sensitivity and allergies are common. May be prone to chronic fatigue syndrome. May suffer from SAD (seasonal affective disorder).

Dietary factors: Likes cold drinks, carbohydrates, and citrus fruits. Dislikes strongly flavored foods.

The Merc. sol. child: Irritating behavior. Shy and cautious. May have a tendency to stammer. Susceptible to ear, nose, and throat ailments.

The Merc. sol. type may be affected by changes in the weather or may suffer from SAD (seasonal affective disorder).

The Nat. mur. type

Appearance: Pear-shaped build in women. Solid, strong-to-lean build in men. Skin can be oily and puffy with a tendency to swell. Red, watery eyes. Dry cracked lips. Medium to dark hair.

Mental and emotional aspects: Prone to suppressing emotions such as fear, loneliness, guilt and anger, which can lead to depression. Suppressed feelings of grief or loss for a loved one or for the self. Can become very despondent and depressed after relationship break-up. May want to cry but cannot. Prone to suffer in silence and not ask for help when needed. Career-minded and successful with a serious outlook on life.

Physical weaknesses: Nervous system. Common problems include: depression; premenstrual

syndrome; anorexia; skin problems; mouth ulcers and cold sores; palpitations and headaches.

Dietary factors: Likes cool drinks, sour and savory foods and craves salt and most carbohydrates. Dislikes coffee and bread.

The Nat. mur. child: Small for their age. Slow development. Well-behaved. Loves animals. Excellent academically but if criticized at school can become very hurt. Can be prone to headaches under pressure.

Nat. mur. types are serious and conscientious. They may be professional and career-minded.

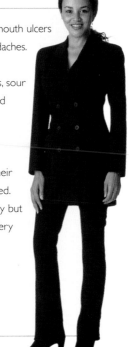

The Nux Vomica Type

Appearance: Slim, particularly when young. Smart appearance. May look stressed and tense. Ages prematurely. Prone to dark circles under the eyes. Face becomes flushed through anger or excitement.

Mental and emotional aspects: Can suffer from addictions and over-indulgence. May have cravings for alcohol, food, and stimulants such as coffee and cigarettes. Can be addicted to sex. Finds it difficult to relax. Can be very ambitious. Impatient. Intolerant and critical and requires perfection in others. The worst thing that can happen to a Nux vomica type is failure.

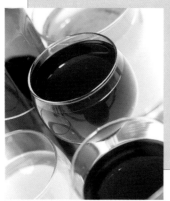

The Nux vomica type may become over-dependent on alcohol or stimulants, which may be craved.

Physical weaknesses: Digestive disorders from hangovers and over-indulgence. Migraines and headaches, hernia, and hay fever. Feels better for sleep.

Dietary factors: Likes fatty and rich food, cheese and cream, alcohol, coffee and spicy foods. Dislikes the effect of some strong spicy foods (despite enjoying eating them).

The Nux vomica child: Irritable and easily bored. May be prone to hyperactivity and ADHD (attention deficit and hyperactivity disorder). May throw tantrums. Competitive as a teenager. Can become addicted to alcohol and drugs, as likes to be rebellious.

The Phosphorus Type

Appearance: Tall and slim with long limbs. Likes to dress well and look stylish. May be artistic and creative in appearance. Fine skin. Can have fair to dark hair.

Mental and emotional aspects: Needs a lot of love and attention. Good fun to be with but can be needy and demanding. Likes to be the center of attraction. Enjoys sympathy when upset or unwell. Expressive, affectionate, and shows emotions easily. Needs reassurance, in particular with looks and body image. Short attention span. Challenging, particularly towards a partner.

Physical weaknesses: Nervous system—in particular fear and hypersensitivity. Circulation problems. Vertigo. Coughs and colds. Weakness of the lungs. Headaches. Prone to left-sided problems.

Dietary factors: Likes salt, spicy food, sour and savory food, carbonated drinks, alcohol, mild cheeses and sweet foods. Dislikes strongly flavored fish and fruit.

The Phosphorus child: Tall and slim with long legs and arms. Nervous. Likes to be with people and center of attention. Loves to receive affection. Strong fear of the dark.

Phosphorus types enjoy mild cheeses. They also enjoy spicy, sour, and savory dishes.

The Pulsatilla Type

Appearance: Can be slightly overweight. Gentle and kind in appearance. Can look younger than actual age. Hair is fair and skin has a rosy complexion. Usually has blue eyes. Blushes easily. Often rests with hands behind the head.

Mental and emotional aspects: Shy and easily embarrassed. Kind and gentle and makes friends easily. Likes to be supported by others. Not assertive and can be indecisive. Cries easily, in particular over cruelty to children and animals, tragic news or weepy movies. Also laughs easily. Avoids confrontation. Loves animals.

Pulsatilla types often rest with their hands behind their head.

Can suppress guilt and anger. Occasionally prone to obsessive or compulsive behavior.

Physical weaknesses: All female reproductive problems. Catarrh. Irritable bowel syndrome. Skin problems. Varicose veins. Styes. Physical symptoms can fluctuate and change rapidly.

Dietary factors: Likes sweet foods, cold foods, and cool drinks. Dislikes fatty foods (particularly cream and butter) and very rich, spicy food.

The Pulsatilla child: Fears the dark and dislikes bedtime. Sensitive to changes in the weather. Becomes tearful and weepy when overtired. Prone to coughs and colds.

The Sepia Type

Appearance: Slim and tall. Often sits with legs crossed. Likes to look attractive and elegant. Medium to dark hair, often with brown eyes.

Mental and emotional aspects: Can be irritable and easily offended. Tendency to be aggressive to loved ones. Cannot handle too much stress and tries to escape pressure and deadlines. Can feel better after weeping, but dislikes it when other people are fussing around. Avoids crowds but fears being alone. Hates being contradicted; holds strong opinions.

Physical weaknesses: These include all menopausal problems. Headaches and migraine. Skin problems. Other common ailments include constipation and hemorrhoids; chronic fatigue syndrome and depression. Conditions usually improve with exertion. Physical problems occur mostly on left side.

Dietary factors: Likes spices, sour and savory food, citrus fruits, sweet foods, and alcohol. Dislikes dairy products, in particular milk, rich and strongly flavored meats, and fatty foods.

The Sepia child: Greedy. Prone to constipation. Can become a bedwetter. Moody. Feels the cold and becomes tired easily. Does not like being alone.

The Sepia type fears being alone but at the same time does not like to be part of a large crowd.

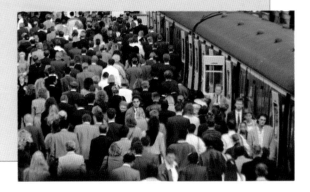

The Silicea Type

Appearance: Often slim or thin, with a large forehead. The head can appear too large for the body. Delicate, fine features—almost doll-like in appearance. The skin of the lips looks gray and can be cracked. The palms of the hand feel sweaty to touch and the nails can be brittle.

Mental and emotional aspects: Appears to have low confidence from a young age. Prone to mental exhaustion. Can become overburdened and overwhelmed. Responsibility weighs heavily upon the Silicea type. Can be indecisive about taking on new projects, moves, and new jobs. Fear of failure may manifest itself as workaholism. Fear of failure

The nails of Silicea types may be rough or brittle. If injured, their skin can take a long time to heal.

can also spread into personal relationships. May stubbornly resist advice from loved ones and friends in order to hide true feelings.

Physical weaknesses: Problems with nervous system, in particular burn-out from new ventures. Exhaustion. Slowness in healing and convalescence. Respiratory illnesses and weaknesses including chest infections and low resistance to coughs and colds. Constipation. Skin problems. Headaches. Feels the cold.

Dietary factors: Likes cold food such as salads and raw vegetables. Dislikes meat and dairy products, in particular cheese and milk. Dislikes very hot food.

The Silicea child: Can be smaller than children of a similar age, with a petite appearance, apart from the head, which may look large for the body size. Feels the cold. Not sporty as has little stamina. Can be shy. Usually tidy and well-behaved.

The Sulfur Type

Appearance: May be slim with poor posture. May look untidy. Hair may be coarse, dry. Skin and lips can be prone to redness.

Mental and emotional aspects: Mind can be cluttered. Can be critical. Likes to argue. May lack willpower and self-esteem. Might not complete ideas or projects.

Physical weakness: Prone to: skin and circulation problems; hemorrhoids and constipation; hot, burning feet; body odor.

Dietary factors: Likes sweet foods, fatty foods, and stimulants such as coffee and chocolate. Likes alcohol, spicy foods, savory foods, citrus fruits, salads, and seafood. Dislikes dairy foods, in particular milk and eggs. Dislikes most hot drinks.

The Sulfur child: Untidy looking. Can be hyperactive in the evening. Does not like bathing, showers or washing hands. Has a very healthy appetite.

The Sulfur type enjoys sour foods such as citrus fruits.

Homeopathic Remedies

In the following pages are details of the main remedies: derivation, treatment use, and tips. Before continuing, read about modalities and get to know the dos and don'ts.

Modalities

Modalities are influences that worsen or improve the symptoms of the patient. They are an invaluable guide to narrowing down the choice of a homeopathic remedy. These are the main types of modality:

• **Physical modalities:** include how the patient is affected by movement, position of the body, touch, rest, exertion, noise, and smells.

• **Temperature:** heat, cold, warmth, wind, damp, and the season of the year may affect the individual's symptoms.

• **Time:** symptoms may be more noticeable in the daytime or at night, or in the morning, afternoon or evening. Symptoms may even change hourly.

• **Diet:** different foods, drinks, stimulants or alcohol may affect the patient and his or her ailment.

• **Localized modalities:** symptoms may be worse on the left or right side of the body. Left-handed and right-handed people may experience symptoms differently.

Dos

• Leave your mouth free from food and liquid 20–30 minutes each side of taking the remedy.
• Use a homeopathic tooth-paste such as calendula, as this will be free from substances that may antidote the remedy.
• Store the remedy in a dark, cool place.
• Check the expiry date before use.
• Keep tablets out of reach of children and pets.
• Store the remedy away from strong-smelling perfumes or essential oils.

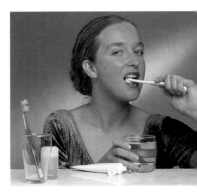

Don'ts

• Don't swallow the tablet; suck it till it dissolves.
• Don't drink coffee or smoke while taking treatment.
• Don't eat mints, peppermints or menthol cough sweets, because this may interfere with the remedy's action. Avoid brushing your teeth with mint or peppermint-flavored toothpaste.
• Don't use the essential oils of camphor, eucalyptus, menthol, peppermint or rosemary.
• Don't touch the pills directly. Always tap the tablets into the lid, because the sweat from your fingertips or palm may absorb the remedy rather than your mouth.
• Don't apply perfume or aftershave 30 minutes either side of taking the remedy.

Aconite

Aconite is derived from Monkshood, a toxic plant used for centuries to treat infections and also to poison arrows for hunting.

Treatment Use

Aconite is useful when any of the following are indicated:

Mental and emotional aspects

● Anxiety and great fear ● Feelings of doom and gloom, especially when accompanied by illness ● A strong fear of death, the dark, and ghosts ● Agoraphobia and panic ● Any form of shock ● Worry and stress about the future ● Nightmares ● Panic attacks ● Vivid imagination ● Unhappiness ● Emotional and physical tension that drains energy from the mind and the body.

Aconite is often used to treat panic attacks. It can also be used when a person is facing any situation that is an ordeal.

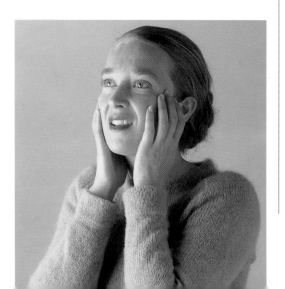

The Monkshood plant (Aconitum napellus) is the source of the remedy Aconite.

Physical aspects

● Headaches with a hot and heavy sensation ● Sore, gritty eyes ● Sore nose, throat or ear problems ● Tightness and pressure around the chest ● Coughs, colds, and influenza ● Sleep problems ● Feelings of restlessness ● Palpitations ● Nervous twitching of the eye ● Sunburn, when accompanied by shaking and fever.

Modalities

● **Better:** for fresh air and warmth.
● **Worse:** in the evening and at night.

Treatment Tips

This remedy is useful for treating ailments that develop suddenly.

This remedy is a useful addition to a homeopathic first aid kit.

Apis Mel.

Apis mel. is derived from the honeybee—the whole bee is used. Propolis, a resin-type substance secreted by bees to repair damage to hive walls, has been used for centuries as a natural antibiotic.

Treatment Use

Apis mel. is useful when any of the following are indicated:

Mental and emotional aspects

- Poor memory • Feelings of jealousy
- Being hard to please • Tearfulness • Apathy and indifference • Constantly complaining and hard to please • Fear of death.

Physical aspects

- Clumsiness • Headaches with a stabbing and stinging pain • Fever with a lack of thirst accompanied by skin that is sensitive to the touch • Itchy, stinging skin • All eye problems that sting and burn • Arthritis when the pain is burning in sensation • Cystitis and other urinary tract infections that cause stinging on passing urine

Apis mel. is often used to help overcome tearfulness.

The remedy from the honeybee provides a range of medicinal substances.

- Insect bites and stings • A constant but spasmodic cough.

Modalities

- **Better:** cool water and a cool room; the application of cold compresses.
- **Worse:** for pressure and touch; heat.

Treatment Tips

Apis mel. is an excellent remedy for treating burning and stinging pain that responds well to being treated with a cool remedy. It is useful for swollen and itchy skin, particularly following insect bites and stings. Useful for any sudden swelling or puffiness of the skin.

This remedy is a useful addition to a homeopathic first aid kit.

Argent. Nit.

Argent. nit. is derived from silver nitrate (a compound of silver). It is poisonous in large amounts. It has a caustic nature and it was used historically to cauterize wounds.

Treatment Use

Argent. nit. is useful when any of the following are indicated:

Silver nitrate crystals are extracted from the mineral acanthite, the main ore of silver.

Mental and emotional aspects

- Apprehension • Fearfulness
- Nervousness • Overactive imagination
- Stage-fright • Phobias, in particular claustrophobia and fear of spiders and insects
- Feeling stressed and in a hurry • Fear of giving talks or addressing groups • Fear of taking examinations.

Physical aspects

- Diarrhea caused by anxiety and tension

• Nightmares • Tight, sore muscles due to constant body tension • Headaches caused by concentrating hard • Flatulence • Trembling and weakness in muscles and limbs • Palpitations and tightness in the chest • Aching, tired eyes • Irritable bowel syndrome.

Modalities

- **Better:** for cool, fresh air and pressure.
- **Worse:** when highly emotional; for concentration; for warmth.

Treatment Tips

A remedy that helps to relieve apprehension and anxiety. Useful when there is fear of a forthcoming event, for example an examination or an interview. Helps control nerves both before and during the event.

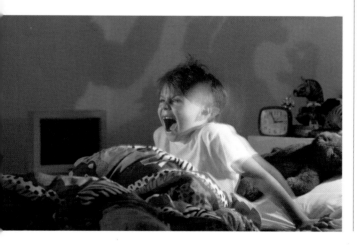

Argent. nit. can be used to help overcome fears and phobias and help with nightmares or an overactive imagination.

Arnica

Arnica is derived from Leopard's Bane, a plant used since the 16th century as a remedy for bruises, muscular aches and pains, and rheumatism.

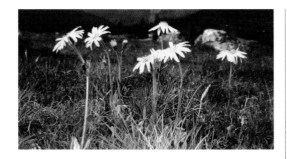

The fresh flowers of the plant Leopard's Bane (Arnica montana) are used to provide a remedy for physical and emotional shock.

- Hot, sensitive, aching headache • Heavy, tired eyes • Concussion • Nosebleeds
- Sore muscles in chest following a bad cough
- Over-exertion • Vertigo.

Modalities

- **Better:** for lying down.
- **Worse:** for moving; cold, damp weather.

Treatment Use

Arnica is useful when any of the following are indicated:

Mental and emotional aspects

- Irritability • Nervousness and oversensitivity • Inability to focus on a task for long • Forgetfulness and indifference
- Agoraphobia • All forms of shock
- Bereavement.

Physical aspects

- Post-surgical convalescence • Labor pains and childbirth • Sore muscles • Swelling
- Bruising • Backache and joint pain
- Sprains • Black eyes • Accidents and falls

Treatment Tips

Arnica is a key remedy for all forms of muscular pain and bruising. It is also very useful applied topically to unbroken skin in a cream or ointment form or as a compress using the tincture. Arnica is one of the most commonly used remedies and is an over-the-counter bestseller.

This remedy is a useful addition to a homeopathic first aid kit.

Arnica is a useful remedy for the physical and emotional impact of childbirth.

Arsen. Alb.

Arsen. alb. is derived from arsenic, which is a metallic poison.

Treatment Use

Arsen. alb is useful when any of the following are indicated:

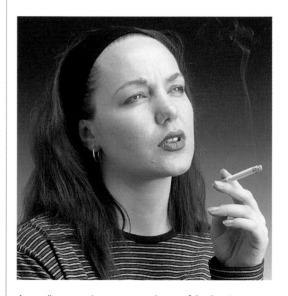

The arsenic compound arsenic trioxide is used to treat a variety of symptoms.

Mental and emotional aspects

- Restlessness ● Anguish and anxiety
- Feelings of hopelessness ● Over-reaction to ailments ● Agitation ● Hypochondria
- Perfectionism demonstrated by obsessive-compulsive behavior ● Inability to cope
- Insecurity ● Fear of the dark ● Fear of poisoning ● Twitches ● Fixed ideas ● Jealousy
- Addictions, including those to alcohol and tobacco ● Fear of being alone ● Fear of death
- Fear of suffocation.

Physical aspects

- Skin, hair and scalp problems, such as psoriasis and dandruff ● Food poisoning
- Vomiting ● Exhaustion ● Headaches
- Mouth ulcers ● Fluid retention ● Mild forms of asthma ● Sore throat, particularly if swallowing is difficult ● Cramp ● Disturbed, restless sleep ● Angina pain.

Modalities

- **Better:** for warm drinks; heat; movement.
- **Worse:** for cold, wet weather.

Treatment Tips

A very useful remedy for the treatment of digestive problems. It is also excellent for treating anxiety and restlessness. It acts on every organ and tissue of the body.

Arsen. alb. acts on the mucous membranes of the digestive tract and respiratory system. It can be used to treat addictions such as smoking.

Aurum Met.

Aurum met. is derived from gold that has first been ground to a powder.

Treatment Use

Aurum met. is useful when any of the following are indicated:

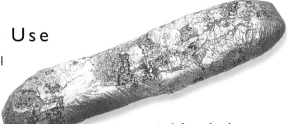

Pure gold ground to a fine powder is used to make Aurum met.

Mental and emotional aspects

● Tendency to become a workaholic ● Prone to perfectionism, leading to dissatisfaction ● Can become deeply upset if criticized ● Extreme unhappiness ● Depression, sometimes leading to suicidal thoughts ● Obsessed with illness and death ● Illness triggered by grief ● Fixed ideas ● Prone to criticize everyone around them ● Cannot always share worries with others, instead brooding on them in isolation ● Prone to nightmares ● Anxiety triggered by loud noises.

Physical aspects

● Illness through depression ● Heart disease, blood and circulatory problems ● Headaches ● Chest pain and breathlessness ● Sinus problems and sinusitis ● Catarrh ● Ear, nose, and throat problems ● Joint pain and skin ulcers ● SAD (seasonal affective disorder).

Modalities

● **Better:** for fresh air and movement.
● **Worse:** for emotional stress and tension; at night; in wintertime.

Treatment Tips

A good remedy to try when others have failed, in particular in cases of depression where there appears to be "no light at the end of the tunnel."

Overwork and stress can be treated by Aurum met. It is used to help many different problems, from depression to heart disease.

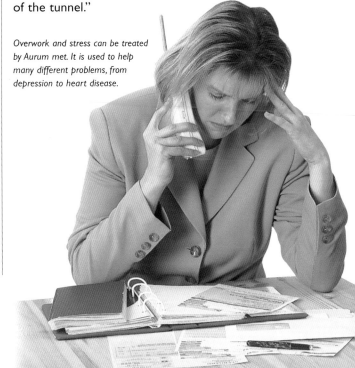

Belladonna

Belladonna is derived from the deadly nightshade plant, which was popular during the Middle Ages for magic rituals.

Treatment Use

Belladonna is useful when any of the following are indicated:

Mental and emotional aspects

• Sudden anger • Feelings of guilt • Stress • Depression triggered by agitation • Sudden temper tantrums and a red face.

Physical aspects

• All pain where there is heat, burning, redness or throbbing • Cold, coughs, and influenza • Sore throats • Earache, made

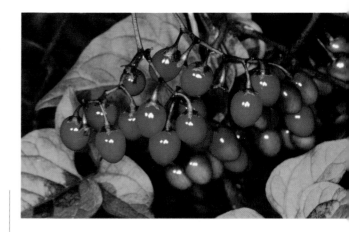

Although every part of the belladonna plant (Atropa belladonna) is poisonous, the leaves and flowers are used in homeopathy.

worse by getting the head wet or cold • Labor pains • Cystitis • All infections that result in inflammation • Teething pain • Boils • Insomnia.

Modalities

• **Better:** for sitting up.
• **Worse:** for noise and movement.

Treatment Tips

An excellent remedy for acute complaints, particularly when accompanied by hot, throbbing sensations.

This remedy is a useful addition to a homeopathic first aid kit.

The remedy Belladonna is used to control sudden anger and violent outbursts of behavior.

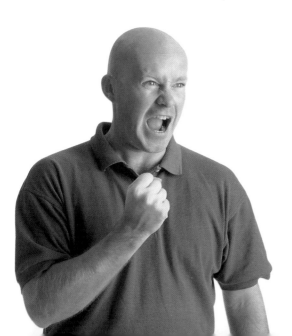

Bryonia

Bryonia is derived from the roots of wild hops grown in central and southern Europe. Bryonia was used by the Romans to treat coughs and wounds.

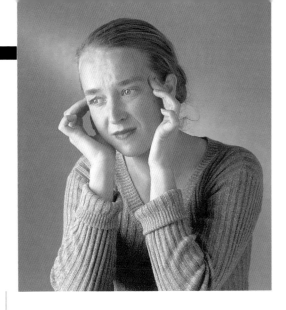

Bryonia is used to treat anger and anxiety, but can also be used as a treatment for violent headaches.

Treatment Use

Bryonia is useful when any of the following are indicated:

Mental and emotional aspects

• Anger, irritability, and restlessness • Poor memory • Fear of death • Prefers to be left alone, particularly when unwell.

Physical aspects

• Headaches with a bursting or splitting sensation • Arthritis and rheumatism • Dry eyes and lips • Very dry and sore throat • Dry, irritating cough • Constipation • Influenza • Pneumonia • Pleurisy with severe chest pain • Colic.

Modalities

• **Better:** for rest and stillness; a cold environment.
• **Worse:** with any kind of movement; cold winds.

Treatment Tips

Best used when there is pain on the slightest movement. Most effective when colds are accompanied by a strong thirst and a very dry throat.

The fresh roots of Bryonia (Bryonia alba) are chopped and pounded to make a pulp for the Bryonia remedy.

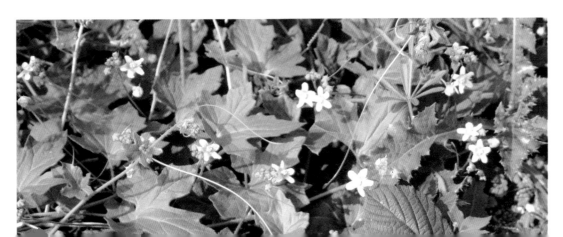

Calc. Carb.

Calc. carb. is derived from calcium carbonate in oyster shells.

Treatment Use

Calc. carb. is useful when any of the following are indicated:

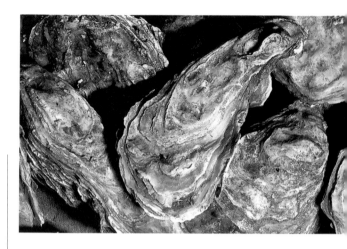

The mother-of-pearl inside oyster shells contains calcium carbonate. This salt is ground to a powder to make this remedy.

Mental and emotional aspects

● Fear of the dark, death, insanity, and impending doom ● In the elderly, fear of a stroke ● Anxiety which can cause palpitations ● Depression with tiredness/lethargy ● Poor memory ● Tiredness and slowness of thought ● Obsession with problems ● Anxiety when criticized ● Hypochondria ● Lowness of spirit● Jealousy ● Laziness ● Fear of disease.

Physical aspects

● Teeth, joint, and bone pain ● Fractures that are slow to heal ● Back pain ● Digestive problems ● Irritable bowel syndrome ● Constipation ● Premenstrual syndrome ● Nasal congestion ● Polyps ● Dry, irritating or tickling coughs ● Obesity ● Eating disorders, in particular bulimia ● Chronic fatigue syndrome ● Warts ● Headaches caused by study or when head feels heavy ● Light-sensitive eyes ● Loss of hearing ● Dark rings around the eyes ● Sour taste in the mouth ● Bleeding gums ● Toothache ● Cramp ● Stiff neck ● Weakness in the knees ● Unhealthy-looking skin.

The Calc. carb. remedy is used to help with anxiety, fear, depression, and feelings of extreme helplessness.

Modalities

● **Better:** for warm weather.

● **Worse:** when cold and damp; for exertion.

Treatment Tips

An excellent remedy for when bones are slow to heal.

Calc. Phos.

Calc. phos. is derived from the mineral salt calcium phosphate.

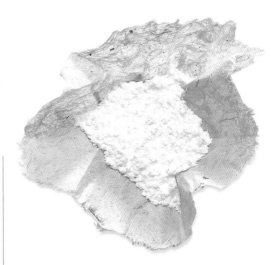

Treatment Use

Calc. phos. is useful when any of the following are indicated:

Mental and emotional aspects

- Unhappiness and discontentment with life, possibly stemming from childhood
- Relationship break-ups may trigger the onset of an illness • Prone to irritability
- Can complain a lot • Tendency to become restless • Difficulty keeping to routines
- In constant need of new things for stimulation • Poor memory.

Physical aspects

- Breaks, fractures, and painful joints • Slow bone or tooth growth in children and teenagers • Exhaustion and fatigue
- Digestive disorders
- Recurrent throat problems.

Modalities

- **Better:** for warm, dry, sunny weather.
- **Worse:** in the cold or damp; for stress and worry.

Calc. phos. is made into a powder through a chemical process.

Treatment Tips

A good remedy if healing is slow or for any bone and joint complaints. It can be used to help "growing pains" in children and adolescents. Good for convalescence.

Calcium phosphate occurs naturally in our teeth, making them hard and rigid. The remedy can be used to treat tooth decay.

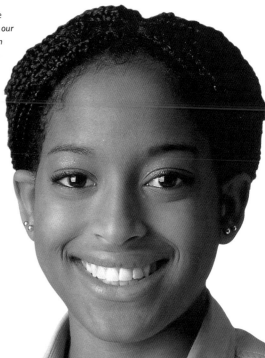

Cantharis

Cantharis is derived from a bright green beetle known as the Spanish fly, which has been known for centuries for its poisonous and irritant properties.

Treatment Use

Cantharis is useful when any of the following are indicated:

Mental and emotional aspects

● Addiction to sex ● Irritability and anger leading to rage and violence ● Screaming with rage ● Severe anxiety.

Physical aspects

● All conditions where there is stinging, burning, itching, and pain ● Cystitis and all urinary tract infections, with pain when urinating ● Burns ● Diarrhea with burning sensation ● Insect stings and bites ● Burning,

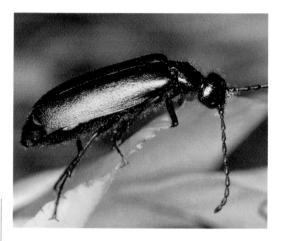

The Spanish fly is the source of the Cantharis remedy. It secretes a substance called cantharidin, which is an irritant.

sore throat ● Sore, stinging eyes ● Hot, aching sensation in the stomach ● Sunburn and inflammation of the skin.

Modalities

● **Better:** for gentle rubbing.
● **Worse:** for touch and movement.

Treatment Tips

Excellent remedy for treatment of cystitis, especially when the condition worsens without warning.

This remedy is a useful addition to a homeopathic first aid kit.

The remedy Cantharis can be used to treat ailments that have burning symptoms, including sunburn.

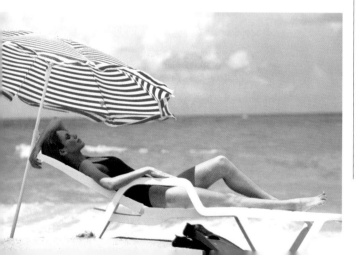

Carbo Veg.

Carbo veg. is derived from vegetable charcoal made from beech, birch or poplar wood. In the past, vegetable charcoal was used to absorb gases to help relieve flatulence.

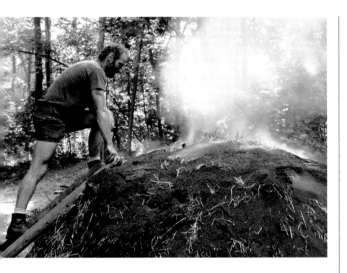

Woods from trees such as beech, birch or poplar are partly burned to make charcoals that have individual properties.

- Indigestion • Flatulence • Feelings of abdominal bloating (even after eating only small amounts) • Headaches after too much food • Headaches with sickness • Coughing • Hoarseness and dryness of the throat • Nosebleeds • Prolonged illness, leaving feelings of exhaustion.

Modalities

- **Better:** for cool, fresh air.
- **Worse:** for fatty foods; in the evening; for lying down.

Treatment Use

Carbo veg. is useful when any of the following are indicated:

Mental and emotional aspects

- Loss of memory • Fear of strangers
- Claustrophobia • Acute shock • Extreme mental exhaustion • Feelings of mental and emotional weakness.

Physical aspects

- Poor circulation • Varicose veins

Treatment Tips

A very good remedy for feelings of overtiredness and being run down. Useful after any operation or illness. Good for speeding a slow recovery. Good for chronic complaints or conditions.

Carbo veg. is mainly given for exhaustion, weakness and lack of energy. It is useful to take following an illness.

Chamomilla

Chamomilla is derived from the whole, fresh chamomile plant. Chamomile has been used for centuries because of its calming, soothing, and healing abilities, particularly in the treatment of skin conditions.

Treatment Use

Chamomilla is useful when any of the following are indicated:

Chamomilla is derived from the juices of the whole, fresh plant (Matricaria recutita) in flower.

Mental and emotional aspects

- Bad temper and anger when unwell
- Irritability and whining • Impatience
- Oversensitivity, which can lead to short-tempered behavior towards loved ones
- Difficult to satisfy.

Physical aspects

- Earache • Toothache
- Insomnia • All skin conditions including eczema • Inflamed skin
- Sleeplessness and colic in children
- Diarrhea • Coughing, particularly at night.

Chamomilla is good for people who suffer from sleeplessness, or who cry out in their sleep because of anxious dreams.

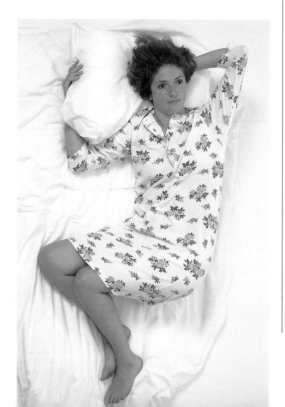

Modalities

- **Better:** for mild weather.
- **Worse:** for heat; for cold winds or fresh air; when angry.

Treatment Tips

Especially good remedy for the treatment of children or babies. Chamomilla is a good bedtime remedy for a baby. Teething problems or colic may cause the baby to cry out and be restless. Chamomilla will help the baby to calm down and sleep.

China

China is derived from Peruvian bark, which contains quinine—one of the first remedies investigated by Samuel Hahnemann.

These leaves are from the Cinchona tree, whose bark contains important remedies.

Treatment Use

China is useful when any of the following are indicated:

Mental and emotional aspects

- Indifference and apathy • Nervous exhaustion • Despair • Fear of creeping, crawling creatures • Outbursts of anger • Spitefulness • Sudden tearfulness • Depression • Eating disorders such as anorexia and bulimia • Lack of concentration • Feelings of being on edge • Hypersensitivity • Alcoholism • Difficulty in self-expression.

Physical aspects

- Loss of body fluid through heat-stroke • Heavy sweating • Fluid retention • Swollen ankles • Headaches • Dizziness • Twitches • Nosebleeds • Tinnitus • Digestive problems including diarrhea and vomiting • Gall bladder complaints

• Feelings of coldness • Shivering • Fatigue, including post-viral exhaustion • Chronic fatigue syndrome • Skin that is sensitive to the touch • Tender scalp.

Modalities

- **Better:** for warmth and sleep.
- **Worse:** for losing bodily fluids; from cold and drafts.

Treatment Tips

A good remedy for burn-out caused by overwork or emotional traumas that produce feelings of exhaustion and weakness. Also a good convalescent remedy.

The China remedy is helpful for irritability and unexpected angry outbursts.

Coffea

Coffea is derived from caffeine: the unroasted coffee bean is used.

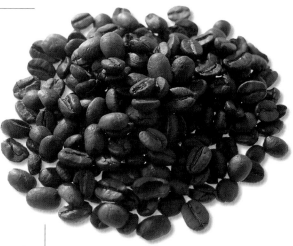

Treatment Use

Coffea is useful when any of the following are indicated:

Mental and emotional aspects

- Hyperactivity and inability to rest the mind
- Insomnia ● Over-excitement in children
- Anxiety and feelings of irritability ● Sensory overload ● Feelings of guilt, particularly over children ● Problems in relationships can cause

Coffea is used to treat overactive mental activity including hyperactivity and over-excitement in children.

Beans roasted for coffee are derived from ripe berries of the Coffea arabica tree. The berries are also used for the Coffea remedy.

physical problems such as headaches and migraines.

Physical aspects

- Sensitive reaction to pain ● Headaches
- Facial pain and neuralgia ● Palpitations brought on by anger or stress ● Skin that reacts in a hypersensitive manner ● Migraine.

Modalities

- **Better:** for warmth.
- **Worse:** for the open air and strong smells.

Treatment Tips

A good remedy for insomnia caused by too much mental activity, particularly when combined with an inability to relax.

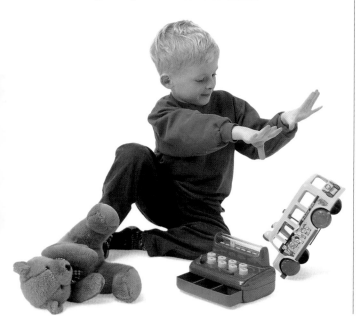

Drosera

Drosera is derived from a tiny plant that traps insects inside its leaves.

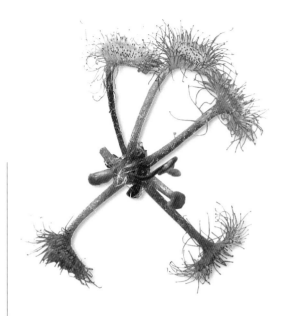

Treatment Use

Drosera is useful when any of the following are indicated:

Mental and emotional aspects

● Feelings of restlessness and anxiety when left alone ● Fear of ghosts ● Difficulty in concentrating ● Sense of persecution ● Prone to talkativeness ● Suspicious of bad or unwelcome news.

Physical aspects

● Colds, especially when accompanied by a violent cough ● Coughs that will not stop and are spasmodic ● Coughs accompanied by nausea or vomiting ● Whooping cough ● Joint pain and growing pains in the legs of teenagers if accompanied by symptoms of stiffness.

Modalities

● **Better:** for being outside in the fresh air and stretching the body and limbs.

● **Worse:** late at night, or lying down for long periods of time; after drinking and eating cold food, after periods of talking.

Drosera rotundifolia is a tiny plant found in bogs and heaths. The whole fresh plant in flower is used for the remedy.

Treatment Tips

An excellent remedy for coughs and colds, in particular for a dry, retching cough.

Drosera is good for joint pain and for "growing pains" of teenagers. The symptoms can be helped by stretching, especially outside.

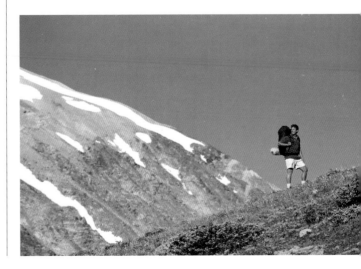

Gelsemium

Gelsemium is derived from the yellow jasmine plant.

Treatment Use

Gelsemium is useful when any of the following are indicated:

Mental and emotional aspects

- Fears and phobias when accompanied by shaking and trembling
- Fear of dentists and doctors ● Fear of being left alone ● Anxiety about forthcoming events, such as meetings
- Drowsiness and confusion ● Panic attacks
- Dislike of insects and creatures that creep and crawl ● Difficulty in sleeping.

Physical aspects

- Influenza ● Sore throat with red tonsils
- Difficulty swallowing ● Fatigue, exhaustion and drowsiness ● Coughs and colds
- Shivering ● Sneezing with a hot and flushed face ● Sore, inflamed eyes ● Migraine and headaches, in particular at the base of the skull or the back of the head ● Weakness and heaviness in the extremities ● Diarrhea that is made worse when anxious.

The climbing plant Carolina jasmine grows in parts of the United States. Its aromatic fresh roots are used in the remedy.

Modalities

- **Better:** for rest and stillness; after going to the toilet.
- **Worse:** for cold, damp weather.

Treatment Tips

The main remedy for influenza. Also excellent for coughs, colds, and sore throats, particularly if accompanied by shivering and fever.

This remedy is a useful addition to a homeopathic first aid kit.

Gelsemium is used for fears and phobias that cause trembling. The remedy works on the spinal cord and respiratory system.

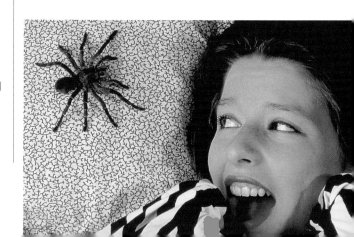

Graphites

Graphites is derived from the mineral graphite or black lead, which is commonly used for pencil leads.

Treatment Use

Graphites is useful when any of the following are indicated:

Mental and emotional aspects

- Fidgeting, in particular when nervous and anxious • Easily triggered feelings of guilt
- Depression • Indecisiveness • Timidness
- Post-menopausal depression • Bulimia.

Physical aspects

- Eczema, particularly behind the knees, on the wrist, inside and outside of ears • Contact dermatitis, particularly on the palms of the hands and between the fingers • Psoriasis
- Dry, cracked, and sore skin • Itchiness or skin eruptions of the scalp • Cold sores
- Stomach problems • Cramp • Constipation
- Styes • Nail problems • Chilblains
- Erratic menstrual cycle • Morning headaches.

Modalities

- **Better:** for eating.
- **Worse:** for heat.

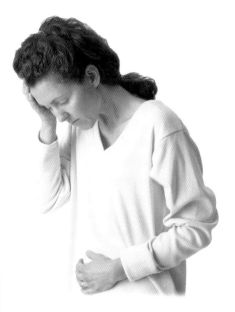

Graphites can be used to treat a wide range of complaints, including stomach problems and morning headaches.

Treatment Tips

Use to treat the first outbreak of skin complaints—in particular eczema and dermatitis, particularly where there is a discharge. In these cases, the remedy should be supported topically with an application of the homeopathic ointment or cream.

This remedy is a useful addition to a homeopathic first aid kit.

Graphite is a carbon, the main constituent of pencils. The mineral graphite is ground into a powder to make the Graphites remedy.

Hamamelis

Hamamelis is derived from the witch-hazel plant. The twigs, bark, and outer layer of the root are used.

Treatment Use

Hamamelis is useful when any of the following are indicated:

Fresh bark, twigs, and the outer root of the witch-hazel plant (Hamamelis virginiana) are ground together and used for the remedy.

Mental and emotional aspects

● Mild depression; the person feels better for being alone ● Irritability and restlessness, particularly in the presence of others.

Physical aspects

● Varicose veins ● Varicocele (varicose veins in the testes) ● Heavy and tired, throbbing and itching, or stinging and aching legs ● Irritated and bloodshot eyes ● Black eyes ● Bruising ● Chilblains ● Nosebleeds ● Mild skin rashes ● Insect bites where accompanied with stinging and aching around the bite ● Mild burns ● Acne and oily skin ● Hemorrhoids.

Modalities

● **Better:** for fresh air; for reading, thinking or talking.
● **Worse:** for warm, damp heat and pressure; for movement.

Treatment Tips

Use at the first sign of varicose veins or hemorrhoids or when these conditions become worse. Treatment can be backed up with a cream or ointment applied directly onto the affected sites.

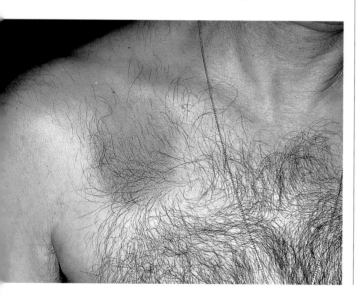

Hamamelis is excellent for both internal and external bleeding. It can be used to treat bruising of the body caused by injury.

Hepar sulf.

Hepar sulf. is derived from
calcium sulfide.

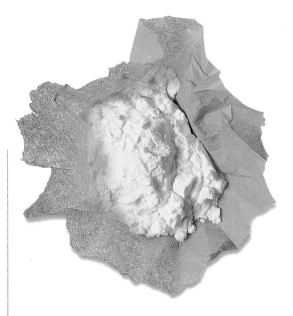

The remedy is prepared chemically by mixing calcium carbonate (derived from oyster shells) together with flowers of sulfur.

Treatment Use

Hepar sulf. is useful when any of the following
are indicated:

Mental and emotional aspects

● Irritation over the slightest matter ● Quick
to take offence ● Talks quickly when anxious
● Over-reacts when angry ● Prone to bouts
of sadness and depression.

Physical aspects

● All skin problems that gather pus and are
slow to heal ● Skin ulcers and bedsores
● Acne and boils ● Earache ● Ear pain with
a sore throat ● Catarrh ● Coughs that create
a hoarse and dry throat ● Cold sores,
particularly around the eyes ● Mouth ulcers
● Influenza with sweating and sneezing
● Cracked, dry lips ● Perspiration that causes
a bad odor, even when deodorant is used.

Modalities

● **Better:** for warmth and for wrapping up
and keeping the head warm.
● **Worse:** for touch and the cold.

Treatment Tips

A good remedy to use when conditions are
slow to heal. Good for clearing infection
and discharges.

The Hepar sulf. remedy can be used to treat infections that cause earache. It helps to expel the discharge from the site of the infection.

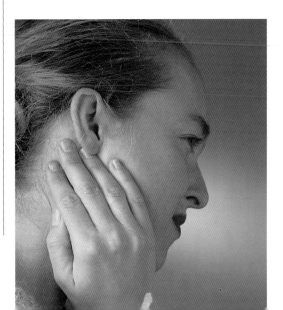

Hypericum

Hypericum is derived from the St John's Wort herb.

Treatment Use

Hypericum is useful when any of the following are indicated:

Mental and emotional aspects

- Depression with tiredness and lethargy
- Depression after surgery or after injury • Vertigo • Shock through injury or emotional trauma
- Stress and anxiety that cause spasms and feelings of tightness in the body.

Physical aspects

- Neuralgia • Puncture wounds received from sharp objects (glass, nails etc) • Splinters
- All wounds and injuries, in particular if crushing is involved • Concussion • Nerve pain or stabbing • Shooting pains • Injuries to the feet, hands and spine • Minor eye injuries • Chronic back pain, with a sensation of pain travelling up and down the back
- Asthma when in a damp environment

The hypericum plant (Hypericum perforatum) produces a red juice from its flowers and leaves, which are used in the remedy.

- Toothache and pain from dental procedures
- Diarrhea • Hemorrhoids with pain and bleeding.

Modalities

- **Better:** for resting the head bent backward; for gentle massage.
- **Worse:** for cold, damp, and foggy weather.

Treatment Tips

A good remedy to use after an injury to the skin, particularly where there is a risk of infection.

This remedy is a useful addition to a homeopathic first aid kit.

Hypericum can be used to treat nerve pain after injury.

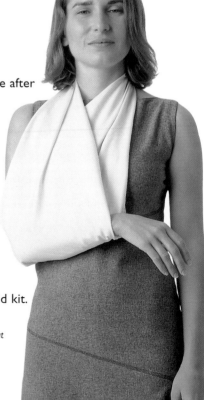

Ignatia

Ignatia is derived from St Ignatius bean, a seedpod from the *Ignatia amara* tree.

Treatment Use

Ignatia is useful when any of the following are indicated:

Mental and emotional aspects

- Highly emotional states • Shock • Anger
- Grief • Inability to express emotions
- Hysteria • Insomnia • Quick, sudden tearfulness • Self-blame and self-pity
- Worry • Sadness over divorce and broken relationships • Sudden, unexpected mood changes • Exhaustion caused by overwork
- Obsessive-compulsive behavior
- Hypochondria • Jealousy • Fixed ideas.

Physical aspects

- Headaches caused by emotional stress and tension • Coughs and sore throats
- Difficulty in swallowing • Twitching of the face triggered by anxiety • Digestive problems, in particular after shock or grief when accompanied with a sinking sensation • Cravings for odd foods when ill
- Diarrhea • Disruptive sleep patterns, particularly if grieving.

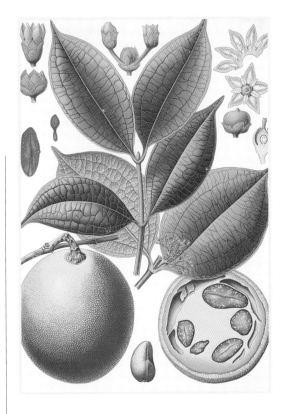

The Ignatia remedy is made from the seeds of the Ignatia amara fruit. The seeds are ground to a powder.

Modalities

- **Better:** for warmth and the sun; change of position.
- **Worse:** in cold air; for emotional upset; in the morning.

Treatment Tips

One of the best remedies for emotional problems. It is good for mood swings, bereavement and any accompanying physical ailments. It is also good if the ailments are very changeable.

Kali phos.

Kali phos. is derived from potassium phosphate.

Treatment Use

Kali phos. is useful when any of the following are indicated:

Mental and emotional aspects

- Complete exhaustion ● Oversensitive reactions and nervousness when stressed
- Frustration due to lack of assertiveness
- Shyness and withdrawal when anxious
- Nervousness when meeting people
- Depression, including post-viral depression
- Nightmares ● Lack of concentration and poor memory ● Fear of a nervous breakdown.

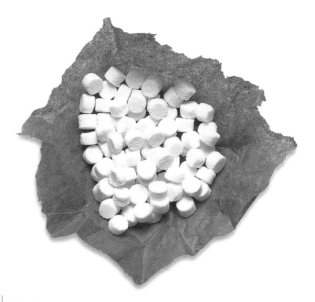

The Kali phos. remedy is prepared chemically from potassium carbonate, derived from potash and dilute phosphoric acid.

Physical aspects

- Weakness of limbs ● Neck and upper back pain ● Tension headaches ● Dizziness after rising from sitting or kneeling ● Chronic fatigue syndrome ● Discharges from colds and catarrh ● Productive coughs ● Diarrhea
- Cystitis.

Modalities

- **Better:** for heat and movement.
- **Worse:** for worry.

Treatment Tips

Known as the "great nerve soother," this is excellent in the treatment of all forms of exhaustion, particularly those brought on by stress.

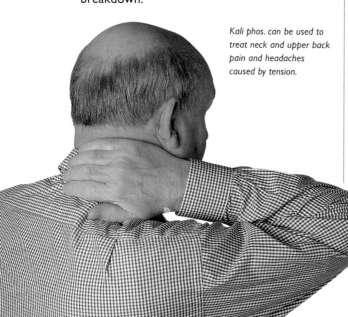

Kali phos. can be used to treat neck and upper back pain and headaches caused by tension.

Lachesis

Lachesis is derived from the venom of the bushmaster snake.

Treatment Use

Lachesis is useful when any of the following are indicated:

Mental and emotional aspects

- Hypersensitivity ● Talkative, rambling, self-absorbed nature ● Restlessness ● Fixed ideas and opinions, in particular about religion
- Fear of personal attack or burglary
- Suspicion of new people ● Jealousy and suspicion of loved ones ● No desire to mix with people ● Suppression of anger
- Nightmares ● Irritability ● Anger after the break-up of relationships ● Addictions, including alcohol, tobacco and drugs
- Premenstrual syndrome ● Post-menopausal depression ● Panic attacks.

Physical aspects

- Headaches, particularly on waking
- Puffy, bloated or swollen face ● Stomach-ache when craving stimulants ● Constrictive, sore throats ● Asthma ● Angina pain
- Palpitations and tightness or constriction of the chest ● Hot flushes ● Bloatedness

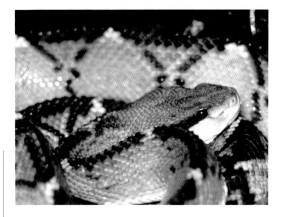

The fresh venom of the bushmaster snake can be dried and made into the remedy.

● Varicose veins ● Hemorrhoids ● Varicocele (varicose veins in the testes) ● Phlebitis and thrombosis ● Menopausal problems.

Modalities

- **Better:** in the open air; for eating and cool drinks.
- **Worse:** when trying to sleep; for touch; for tight clothing

Treatment Tips

Excellent for all circulatory problems. Also good for extreme stress when accompanied with pains and tightness in the chest.

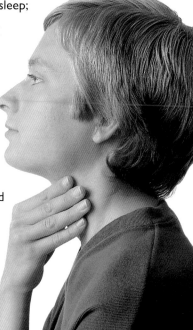

Swollen, sore throats are helped by Lachesis, which eases the pain and makes it easier to take in fluids that were previously difficult to swallow.

Ledum

Ledum is derived from the
wild rosemary plant.

Treatment Use

Ledum is useful when any of the following
are indicated:

Mental and emotional aspects

- Sleep disturbance with night sweats
- Impatience • Timidness.

Physical aspects

- Feelings of hotness and swelling
triggered by stress • Wounds
- Stings with bruising and
puffiness • Grazes and cuts • Bites
- It can prevent cuts, bites or stings from
becoming infected • Injury to the eyes
- Arthritic and rheumatic pain affecting the
ankles, knees or lower legs • Hot, burning
sensations in the limbs • Gout.

Modalities

- **Better:** for cold compresses.
- **Worse:** at night; with heat.

*The Ledum remedy can be
used to help alleviate night
sweats and sleeplessness.*

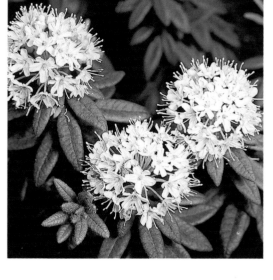

*Fresh, flowering wild rosemary plants (Ledum palustre) are dried
and powdered to make the remedy.*

Treatment Tips

This is an ideal remedy for puncture wounds.
It can prevent any infection caused through
bites, stings, and cuts.

This remedy is a useful addition
to a homeopathic first aid kit.

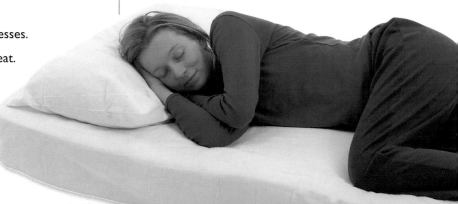

Lycopodium

Lycopodium is derived from the pollen dust of an evergreen herb.

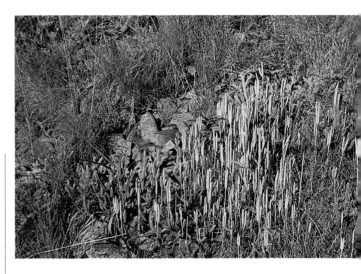

The flowering spikes of the lycopodium herb provide yellow pollen dust, which is shaken out of the plant and used for the remedy.

Treatment Use

Lycopodium is useful when any of the following are indicated:

Mental and emotional aspects

- Lack of self-confidence ● Sexual fears
- Anxiety and fear of interviews and speeches
- Sensitivity ● Forgetfulness ● Irritation caused by minor matters ● Dislike of being contradicted ● Feelings of stress when meeting strangers ● Fear of ghosts, death, and the dark ● Dislike of being alone
- Suppression of fears ● Agoraphobia
- Chronic fatigue syndrome ● Nervous breakdown ● Bulimia.

Physical aspects

- Digestive disorders including indigestion, irritable bowel syndrome, nausea, ulcers, hunger pains, feeling bloated after little food, flatulence, constipation ● Impotence
- Sore throats ● Dry cough
- Extreme tiredness followed by colds or influenza ● Bladder and kidney problems, including kidney stones ● Prostate problems ● Hair loss ● Restless legs at night ● Cold hands and feet ● Headaches over the eyes ● Shoulder pain ● Varicose veins ● Chronic eczema.

Modalities

- **Better:** for small meals and movement.
- **Worse:** for heat and stuffy environment.

Treatment Tip

The first remedy to use for digestive disorders.

The Lycopodium remedy helps cure digestive complaints, particularly indigestion.

Merc. Sol.

Merc. sol. is derived from the black oxide of mercury.

Treatment Use

Merc. sol. is useful when any of the following are indicated:

Mental and emotional aspects

- Slowness and sluggishness of thought
- Distrust of others • Fear of burglary and abuse • Poor memory and difficulty in recall
- Mental and emotional weakness and fatigue
- Chronic fatigue syndrome • Restlessness and anxiety • Deep insecurity
- Suspiciousness • Sensitivity to criticism
- Quick, sudden and aggressive temper
- Lack of willpower • Tendency to be arrogant • Emotional repression.

Physical aspects

- Stammering • Dribbling from the mouth

Liquid mercury is dissolved in dilute nitric acid, forming a gray-black precipitate. This is used to make the remedy.

when sleeping • Tiredness in the limbs and feelings of weakness through the whole body • Body odor
- Cutting, burning pains • Gum and mouth problems • Mouth ulcers
- Bad taste in the mouth, in particular a metallic taste • Oral thrush • Sore throats
- Cold sores • Conjunctivitis with discharge
- Spasmodic coughs • Joint pain • Catarrh
- Scalp problems, eruptions, and crustiness of the scalp • Bed sores.

Modalities

- **Better:** for rest in moderate temperatures.
- **Worse:** at night; for heat or changes in temperature.

Treatment Tips

An excellent remedy for problems with the mouth, especially mouth ulcers and gum problems.

Merc. sol. can be used to treat mouth and throat complaints, including gingivitis, halitosis, and tonsillitis.

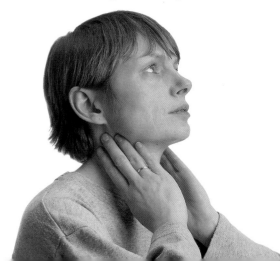

Natrum mur.

Natrum mur. is derived from a mineral rock salt called sodium chloride.

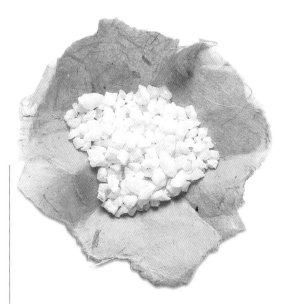

Treatment Use

Natrum mur. is useful when any of the following are indicated:

Mental and emotional aspects

- Anxiety and depression caused by suppressed grief • Repressed fear
- Agoraphobia • Fear of thunderstorms
- Hypochondria • Agitation • Guilt
- Anorexia • Shock • Low self-worth
- Premenstrual syndrome • Quick changing of emotions without warning • Resentment
- Tendency to sulk or keep feelings locked up.

Physical aspects

- Sunstroke • Migraine • Eye strain
- Cold sores • Cracked and dry lips
- Mouth ulcers • Inflamed gums • Boils and warts • Anemia • Constipation • Backache
- Irregular periods • Hair loss • Oily skin and hair • Coughs and colds • Palpitations.

Modalities

- **Better:** for cool, fresh air.
- **Worse:** for heat and sunlight; on waking.

Rock salt is the source of this remedy. It is formed by the evaporation of salty water, which leaves a thick, salty crust behind.

Treatment Tips

A good remedy for people who brood on the past. Very good for treating emotional trauma, such as anxiety or depression caused by loss, grief or separation.

The Natrum mur. remedy may help a fear of thunderstorms. Symptoms of anxiety may be made worse by thundery weather.

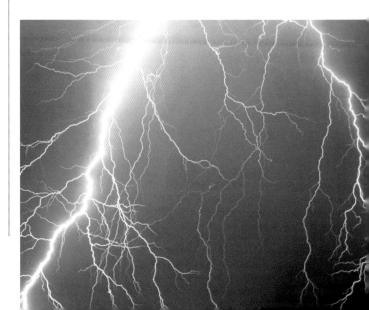

Nux vomica

Nux vomica is derived from the poison strychnine, which is extracted from the seeds of the *Strychnos nux vomica* tree.

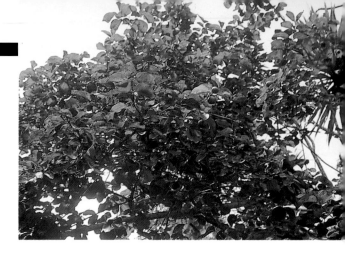

The leaves, bark, and seeds of the Strychnos nux vomica *tree all contain strychnine, but it is usually extracted from the dried seeds.*

Treatment Use

Nux vomica is useful when any of the following are indicated:

Mental and emotional aspects

● Tendency to over-indulge ● Cravings for stimulants such as alcohol, tobacco, and rich foods ● Addictive nature ● Fear of failure ● Argumentative ● Critical ● Fear of spiders and beetles ● Dread of death ● Depression ● Insomnia ● Hyperactivity ● Frustration.

Physical aspects

● Digestive problems, such as indigestion and heartburn ● Food poisoning ● Vomiting ● Constipation ● Diarrhea ● Stomach cramps ● Lower back pain ● Hiccups ● Headaches and migraines ● Hay fever ● Colds and influenza ● Blocked nose ● Heavy, aching muscles ● Fragility ● Morning sickness and cramp in pregnancy.

Modalities

● **Better:** for sleep.
● **Worse:** in the morning.

Treatment Tips

Excellent "hangover" remedy. Also good for aiding digestion and promoting the appetite.

This remedy is a useful addition to a homeopathic first aid kit.

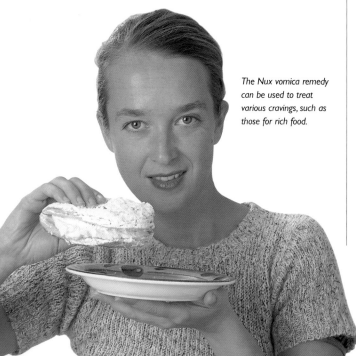

The Nux vomica remedy can be used to treat various cravings, such as those for rich food.

Phosphorus

Phosphorus is derived from a mineral found in phosphates and living matter. It's found in bones, teeth, and bodily fluids.

Treatment Use

Phosphorus is useful when any of the following are indicated:

Mental and emotional aspects

- Hypersensitivity • Excessive imagination
- Easily angered • Fear of darkness and death
- Suppression of fear • Fixed ideas • Fatigue
- Craving for reassurance • Unnecessary worry about health • Nightmares and insomnia • Facial twitches • Shock
- Low spirits • Clairvoyant episodes
- Preference for company and fear of loneliness.

Physical aspects

- Unproductive, hard, dry cough with a tight, heavy chest • Low resistance to infections
- Sore throat with hoarseness • Pneumonia
- Bronchitis • Feels the cold • Asthma
- Bruising • Nose bleeds • Bleeding gums
- Heavy periods • Headaches • Vertigo
- Styes • Panic attacks • Exhaustion and fatigue • Food poisoning • Heartburn

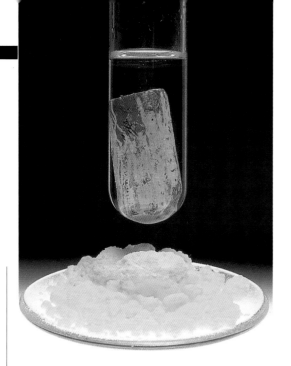

Phosphorus is a yellowish non-metallic mineral, derived from phosphates and living matter.

- Back pain with a burning, hot sensation
- Dandruff • Weakness in the extremities.

Modalities

- **Better:** for warm, fresh air; touch and rubbing.
- **Worse:** for over-exertion; at night.

Treatment Tips

This is the ideal remedy for relieving ailments that are triggered by fear and anxiety as it helps to soothe the nervous system.

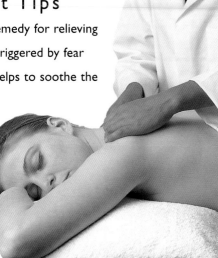

The symptoms helped by the Phosphorus remedy may be further alleviated by massage or rubbing.

Pulsatilla

Pulsatilla is derived from the pulsatilla plant, which is native to Scandinavia, Denmark, Germany, and Russia. The fresh plant in flower is used.

Treatment Use

Pulsatilla is useful when any of the following are indicated:

Mental and emotional aspects
● Tendency to burst into tears without warning ● Quiet temperament ● Suppression of fear ● Depression ● Obsessive-compulsive behavior ● Fear of the opposite sex ● Fear of the dark and ghosts ● Very tearful when grieving ● Bulimia.

Physical aspects
● Coughs and colds
● Runny nose ● Catarrh
● Conjunctivitis
● Digestive problems
● Irritable bowel syndrome ● All menstrual and menopausal problems, particularly if accompanied

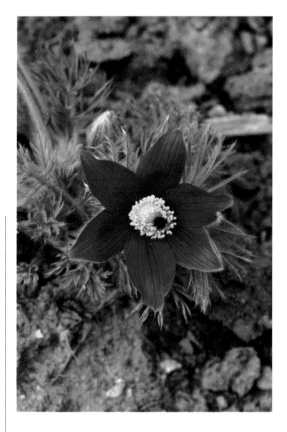

The flowers of pulsatilla plant Pulsatilla nigricans are crushed for their juices, which are used to make the remedy.

by depression ● Lower back pain
● Headaches ● Varicose veins ● Arthritis
● Styes ● Incontinence ● Skin problems.

Modalities
● **Better:** for crying and sympathy; cool, fresh air; gentle exercise.
● **Worse:** for heat; for rich or fatty foods.

Treatment Tips
This remedy works well on the mental state of the individual.

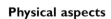
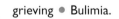

The Pulsatilla remedy is useful for depression and weepiness.

R h u s   t o x .

Rhus tox. is derived from the fresh
leaves of the poison ivy plant.

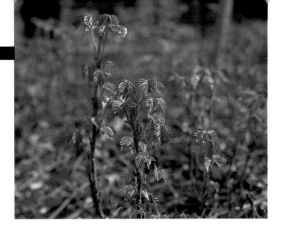

*The leaves are collected from the poison ivy plant before
it flowers and are pulped to make the remedy.*

Treatment Use

Rhus tox. is useful when any of the following
are indicated:

Mental and emotional aspects

● Irritability ● Depression ● Suicidal thoughts
● Lack of joy in life ● Anxiousness ● Fear of
being poisoned ● Anxiety at night.

Physical aspects

● Skin problems, including eczema, dermatitis
and blistering ● Burning, itching, swollen skin
● Cold sores ● Nappy rash ● Sciatica
● Chicken pox ● Shingles ● Influenza
● Sore, stinging eyes ● Muscular aches and
pains ● Stiffness ● Joint pain ● Back pain
● Arthritis and rheumatism ● Sprains and
strains ● Jaw pain ● Frozen shoulder
● Neuralgia ● Post-operative recovery
● Repetitive strain injury.

Modalities

● **Better:** for movement; for a warm,
dry atmosphere.
● **Worse:** for rest and stillness; for cold,
damp weather.

Treatment Tips

This is an excellent remedy for muscular aches
and pains. Eczema and other skin problems
often respond to this remedy when others fail.

This remedy is a useful addition
to a homeopathic first aid kit.

*The Rhus tox. remedy may help repetitive strain injury, which can
be caused by spending long hours using a computer keyboard.*

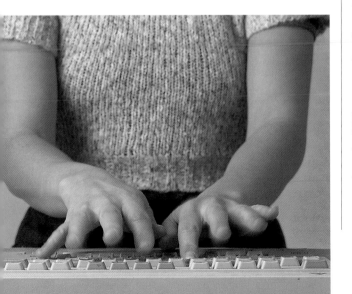

Ruta grav.

Ruta grav. is derived from the *Ruta graveolens* herb. The juice from the whole plant is used, before the plant flowers.

Treatment Use

Ruta grav. is useful when any of the following are indicated:

Mental and emotional aspects

• Low personal satisfaction
• Depression • Critical of others and self • Anxiety.

Physical aspects

• Aches and pains in bones and muscles • Deep, aching pain
• Arthritis and rheumatism • Lower back pain, where the pain feels deep and penetrating • Repetitive strain injury
• Injuries to ligaments, tendons and cartilage
• Sciatic pain • Chest and rib pain caused by coughing • Eye strain and exhaustion from overwork • Headaches, in particular from reading • Constipation.

Modalities

• **Better:** for movement.
• **Worse:** for cold, damp weather; lying down.

Juice is extracted from the whole plant (Ruta graveolens) before it flowers.

Treatment Tips

This remedy acts upon the periosteum (the lining of the bone) and cartilage, so it is excellent for injuries to gliding joints such as the ankle and wrist. This remedy is also the first choice for repetitive strain injury—an inflammation of the tendon sheaths of the arm and wrist.

Ruta grav. can be used for deep aching pain and rheumatism. Damp weather can make the symptoms of such conditions worse.

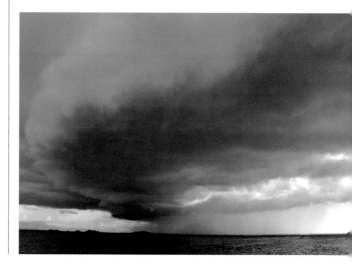

S e p i a

Sepia is derived from the ink of the cuttlefish.

Treatment Use

Sepia is useful when any of the following are indicated:

Mental and emotional aspects

- Menopausal depression
- Exhaustion and slowness of thought • Feelings of weakness • Tendency to cry easily • Stress and anxiety • Feelings of being unable to cope
- Fear of sickness and disease • Fixed ideas
- Irritability • Grief, particularly on separation or relationship break-ups.

Physical aspects

- Chronic fatigue syndrome
- Menopausal problems, including hot flushes and night sweats • Ovarian, vaginal, and

The Sepia remedy can be used to treat hot flushes during the menopause.

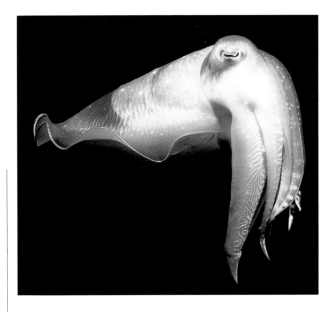

The cuttlefish squirts a dark ink for its protection. The pigments from the ink are used to make the remedy.

uterine complaints, including prolapse of the uterus • Heavy periods • Thrush • Backache
- Flatulence and abdominal and stomach tenderness • Headaches and migraines
- Constipation • Hemorrhoids and varicose veins • Hair loss • Tiredness • Dizziness
- Sweaty feet.

Modalities

- **Better:** for sleep; warmth; gentle exercise.
- **Worse:** in the morning; for a sedentary lifestyle.

Treatment Tips

An excellent remedy for women, because it helps greatly with menopausal problems. It is also good for exhaustion.

Silicea

Silicea is derived from the main part of most rocks and plant stems. It is also found in teeth, hair, and bones. This remedy is mainly derived from quartz or flint.

Rock crystal is a type of quartz. Traditionally, quartz or flint have been used to prepare the remedy.

Treatment Use

Silicea is useful when any of the following are indicated:

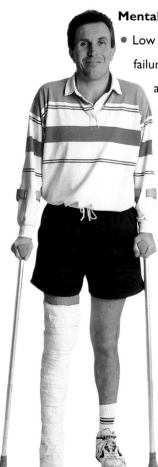

The Silicea remedy can be used for helping fractured bones to heal.

Mental and emotional aspects

● Low self-confidence ● Fear of failure ● Lack of assertiveness and timidity ● Anxiety about important events ● Exhaustion after periods of concentration ● Performance fear ● Obsessiveness about detail ● Stubbornness ● Fear of commitment.

Physical aspects

● Weak immune system ● Weak nervous system ● Slowness of healing, particularly broken bones and fractures ● Recurrent coughs, colds, and respiratory infections ● Ear infections ● Sore, throbbing throat ● Swelling of glands ● Catarrh ● Chest infections, especially if a family history of tuberculosis ● Boils ● Headaches, especially if triggered by cold ● Painful joints and bones ● Anorexia and under-nourishment in general ● Unhealthy skin, including acne ● Slow bone growth in babies and children ● Light-sensitive eyes ● Poor sense of smell ● Cracking at the corner of the mouth ● Sensitive gums ● Constipation ● Sweaty feet and head.

Modalities

● **Better:** for keeping warm.

● **Worse:** for cold, damp weather; drafts.

Treatment Tips

A good remedy to use if an individual has low resistance to disease and is slow to recover from infection.

Staphysagria

Staphysagria is derived from the seed of the plant sometimes known as stavesacre or palmated larkspur. It was used by the Greeks and Romans as a remedy.

Treatment Use

Staphysagria is useful when any of the following are indicated:

Mental and emotional aspects

- Suppression of emotions, in particular anger
- Outbursts of temper • Fixated about an illness, symptom or emotional problem
- Likes to be alone • Sensitive to criticism and easily offended • Resentment and jealousy • Hypersensitivity • Sex addiction
- Workaholic • Over-indulgence in alcohol, tobacco or food.

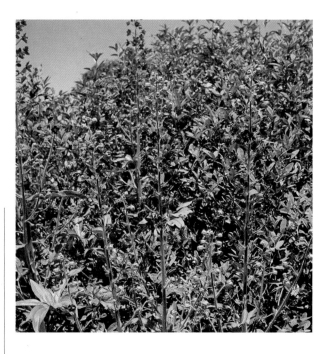

The seeds of the Delphinium staphysagria *plant are used to make the remedy.*

Physical aspects

- Post-operative trauma • Enlargement of prostate gland • Skin problems • Headaches
- Flatulence • Teething problems • Neuralgia
- Styes • Inflammation of the eyes

Modalities

- **Better:** for warmth.
- **Worse:** for suppressing emotions; touch.

Treatment Tips

It can be used to treat suppressed emotions and anger and diseases stemming from these.

The remedy Staphysagria can be used to control suppressed rage.

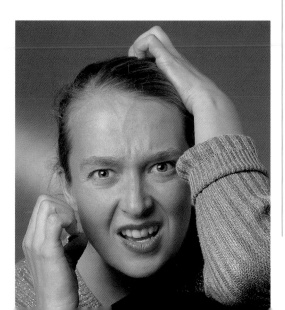

Sulfur

Sulfur is derived from the mineral sulfur.

Treatment Use

Sulfur is useful when any of the following are indicated:

A powder called flowers of sulfur is extracted from the mineral sulfur and used to make the remedy.

Mental and emotional aspects

- Forgetfulness • Inability to think clearly • Lack of for others • Laziness • Irritability • Self-centeredness and selfishness • Argumentative • Aggressive tendencies • Claustrophobia • Fear of heights (vertigo) • Fear of oppression • Bulimia • Insomnia • Post-menopausal depression • Alcoholism • Addiction to smoking • Lack of willpower • Nightmares.

Physical aspects

- Burning, itching skin • Eczema, dermatitis, psoriasis • Thrush • Diaper rash • Catarrh • Hot, sweaty burning feet • Digestive disorders • Constipation • Diarrhea •Indigestion • Loss of appetite • Hemorrhoids • Lower back pain • Gout • Headaches • Conjunctivitis • Red, sore, and itchy eyes • Offensive body odor • Menopausal problems such as hot flushes and dizziness • Hair loss • Dry, itchy scalp • Dry lips • Sore throats • Stiff knees and ankles.

Modalities

- **Better:** for warm, fresh air.
- **Worse:** early mornings and late nights; damp, cold weather; washing; prolonged sitting and standing.

Treatment Tips

Skin problems, particularly where the skin is red and itchy (such as eczema), respond well to this remedy. It is also a good general remedy for detoxification.

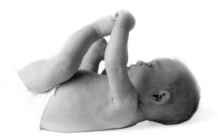

The remedy Sulfur can be used to treat skin conditions such as diaper rash.

Thuja

Thuja is derived from the leaves and twigs of the evergreen conifer tree, which is commonly known as the white cedar tree.

Treatment Use

Thuja is useful when any of the following are indicated:

Mental and emotional aspects

- Anorexia • Distorted ideas of body image
- Fear of strangers • Facial twitches • Fixed ideas • Anxiety • Cries easily • Dyslexia
- Paranoia • Interrupted sleep • Lack of self-esteem • Secretive • Manipulative but weak.

Physical aspects

- Warts • Verrucas • Skin complaints
- Very oily skin • Acne • Perspiration with odor • Headaches • Polyps of the nose
- Styes • Nail problems • Hemorrhoids
- Loss of appetite • Constantly cold
- Urethral and vaginal infections • Menstrual problems including cramps.

Modalities

- **Better:** for movement.
- **Worse:** for cold and damp; at night.

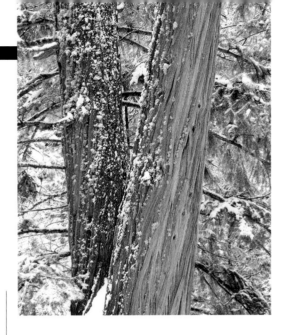

The leaves and twigs of the arborvitae conifer (Thuja occidentalis) are pounded to make the remedy.

Treatment Tips

Thuja is the first remedy of choice for dealing with warts and verrucas. In addition, it can be applied topically to provide back-up to the oral treatment.

In addition to its use in dealing with warts, verrucas, and other skin complaints, Thuja remedy can be used to combat loss of appetite.

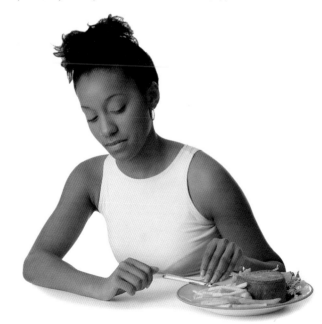

Zinc. Met.

Zinc. met. is derived from zinc.

Treatment Use

Zinc. met. is useful when any of the following are indicated:

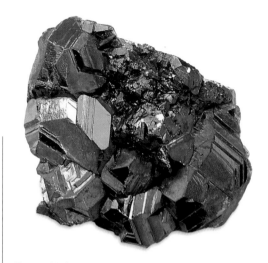

Zinc is a bluish metal; it is ground up to make the powder from which the remedy is made.

Mental and emotional aspects

- Mental fatigue • Poor memory
- Restlessness • Depression • Alcoholism
- Irritability • Jumpiness • Constant fidgeting.

Physical aspects

- Exhaustion • Restless legs • Tiredness through lack of sleep • Weakness and exhaustion • Head feels heavy • Chilblains • Cramp • Varicose veins • Chronic fatigue syndrome • Bulimia • Sensitivity to noise • Anemia.

Modalities

- **Better:** for bowel movement; emotional reassurance.
- **Worse:** after food.

Treatment Tips

A good remedy for lack of vitality or for treating exhaustion. It is also good for constant feelings of coldness.

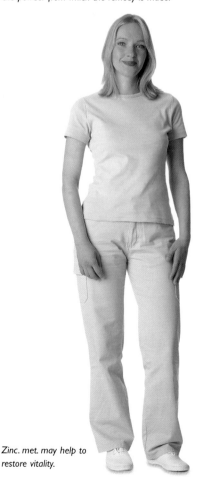

Zinc. met. may help to restore vitality.

Topical Applications

Some homeopathic remedies can be used in preparations that are applied directly to the skin. These are known as topical applications and are an ideal way to back up the oral remedies. They can also be used on their own or as a first aid treatment. Topical treatments come in the forms listed below.

Forms of Topical Treatments

Creams: Easily absorbed.

Ointments: Greasier than creams in texture; best for larger areas.

Tinctures: Liquid remedies ready for dilution in water; best for cuts and grazes. Dilute according to instructions.

Massage balms: Remedies in vegetable oil base, ready for massage.

Sprays: Ready-mixed; useful for insect bites and stings (eg, pyrethrum spray).

The following remedies are the most widely available topical applications and are listed with the conditions they are usually used to treat.

Arnica: Bruising. Muscular aches and pains. Sprains and strains. After sport or exercise. Joint pain. Aching and stiff back. Tired, aching feet. First signs of repetitive strain injury. Frozen shoulder. Neck pain and stiffness. Sunburn (but do not apply to broken skin).

Calendula: Sensitive, dry, irritated, cracked and inflamed skin. Acne. Contact dermatitis. Eczema. Rashes. Cradle cap. Cold sores. Razor burn. Sunburn. Can be used on babies for minor irritations such as diaper rash and grazes. Good for cleaning cuts and wounds. Can be used as a facial moisturizer or aftershave balm.

Graphites: Eczema. Contact dermatitis. Psoriasis. Varicose eczema, or to help prevent it where skin is dry, thin and translucent. Extremely dry, itchy, sore skin. Sore skin in and around the nose accompanied by a cold. Cold sores. Use as a facial moisturizer to help clear eczema, dermatitis or allergic reaction to cosmetics.

Hamamelis: Sore, burning, itching skin. Varicose veins. Phlebitis. Hemorrhoids. Heavy, aching legs and feet, in particular after long periods of standing. *Always apply lightly around varicose sites. Do not use on broken skin.*

Hypericum: Cuts, sores, wounds, scrapes, and grazes. Cold sores. Itchy, irritated, and inflamed skin. Splinters. Nail irritations (nail-bed cuts or bitten, sore nails). Cracked, sore lips. Blisters. Sore, bleeding hemorrhoids.

Rhus tox.: Muscular aches and pains, in particular from physical over-exertion. Repetitive strain injury. Joint pain, including tennis elbow and knee injuries. Arthritis and rheumatism. Sciatica. Useful to use after Arnica, once the bruising has diminished. *Do not apply to broken skin.*

Ruta grav.: Stiffness and pain in tendons, ligaments, joints, and muscles where there is a deep aching. Repetitive strain injury. Sciatica. Rib and chest pain brought on by coughs. Good for sports-related ankle and wrist pain. *Do not apply to broken skin.*

Thuja: Warts. Verrucas. Brittle, weak nails.

First Aid and Travel Kit

 A homeopathic first aid kit is a very useful item to have around the house, in the car or on vacation. Make sure it is readily available. You may wish to purchase a remedy box in which to store your first aid kit.

Several homeopathic pharmacies and suppliers provide a ready-made first aid kit. Some of these consist of up to 18 remedies in small bottles or vials. It may not be necessary for you to have this many remedies. Look at the remedies listed in this book and decide which ones would be most useful. You may have already used some of the remedies or have worked out your constitutional remedy, and therefore know which ones work well for you.

KIT REMEDIES

The following ten remedies would normally be enough to treat most first aid situations.

Aconite

Panic. Fear. Pain. First signs of a cold or sore throat and fever. Inability to relax. Anxiety. To help induce sleep after a long journey. Any condition with a sudden onset.

Apis mel.

For bites and stings. Fluid retention and swelling. Swelling of legs and feet with travel.

Arnica

Shock. Injury. Bruising. Neck, back, shoulder, and joint pain. Sprains and strains. Headaches. Jet lag. Topical application of Arnica cream or ointment can be used for bruising, sprains, strains, and sunburn (but not on broken skin).

Cantharis

Chronic cystitis. Burning, stinging pain. Insect bites and stings. Sunburn.

Gelsemium

Sore throats. Coughs and colds. Influenza with shivering.

Graphites

Allergies. Reactions or break-outs of the skin due to change of climate or change of washing powders. Reactions to swimming pool chemicals. Eczema. Dermatitis. Topical application of Graphites cream can be used to soothe eczema, dermatitis or itchy, irritated skin.

Hypericum/Calendula mixture

Tincture for cleaning cuts and wounds. Ointment or cream for application on wounds, cuts, and grazes or insect bites and stings.

Ledum

Puncture wounds. Splinters. Bites and stings.

Nux vomica

Food poisoning. Travel sickness. Upset stomach. Jet lag. Hangover. Over-indulgence in rich foods.

Rhus tox.

Muscular aches and pains. Stiffness and over-exertion. Back and joint pain. Muscular aches and pain. Useful after skiing, trekking or activity holidays. The topical application of Rhus tox. can be used for muscular aches and pains, after sport or other exertion.

Useful Addresses

Please note that some homeopaths prefer not to have their address or telephone number listed on registers. Always check the qualifications of your homeopath. Personal recommendation is always the best way to find a good homeopath, but the following organizations may also help:

Homeopathic Organizations

American Association of Homeopathic Pharmacists
P.O. Box 2273
Falls Church, VA 22042

American Institute of Homeopathy
1500 Massachusettes Ave.,
NW Washington, D.C. 20005

Foundation for Homeopathic Education and Research
2124 Kittredge St.
Berkeley, CA 94704
(510) 649-8930

National Center for Homeopathy
801 North Fairfax St.
Suite 306
Alexandria, VA 22314
(703) 548-7790

International Foundation for Homeopathy
2366 Eastlake Ave.,
No.301 Seattle, WA 98102
(206) 324-8230

American Board of Homeotherapeutics
1500 Massachusetts Ave., NW
Washington, D.C. 20005

If you have trouble obtaining your remedy from a local pharmacist, or health store, then try the suppliers below. Most will supply ointments, creams, and tinctures as well as the homeopathic tablets, boxes, and carry cases.

Suppliers of Homeopathic Medicines

Standard Homeopathic Company
P.O. Box 61607
436 W. Eighth Street
Los Angeles, CA 90014
(213) 321-4284

Washington Homeopathic Pharmacy
4914 Del Ray Ave.
Bethesda, MD 20814
(301) 656-1695

Luyties Pharmacal Co.
4200 Laclede Ave.
St. Louis, MO 63108
(800) 325-8080

Dolisos America, Inc.
3014 Rigel Ave.
Las Vegas, NV 89102
(702) 871-7153

Humphreys Pharmacal Co.
63 Meadow Road
Rutherford, NJ 07070
(201) 933-7744

Weleda, Inc.
841 South Main Street
Spring Valley, NY 10977

Homeopathic Educational Services
2124 Kittredge St.
Berkeley, CA 94704
(510) 649-0294

Boericke and Tafel, Inc.
2381 Circadian Way
Santa Rosa, CA 95407
(707) 571-8202

Boiron-Borneman
1208 Amosland Road
Norwood, PA 19074
(215) 532-2035

Biological Homeopathic Industries (BHI)
11600 Cochiti S.E.
Albuquerque, NM 87123
(800) 621-7644

Hahnemann Pharmacy
828 San Pablo
Albany, CA 94706
(510) 527-3003

Weinstock Brauer Pharmaceuticals, Inc.
100 East Thousand Oaks Blvd., Suite 265
Thousand Oaks, CA 91360
(805) 495-6704

Index